# I've Lost My Mum

*Disclaimer*

*This book is designed to provide helpful information on the sub-jects discussed. It is general reference information which should not be used to diagnose any medical problem and is not intended as a substitute for consulting with a medical or professional practitioner. Some names and identifying details have been changed to protect the privacy of the individuals.*

# I've Lost
# My Mum

*Cassandra Farren*

Published in 2019 by Welford Publishing
Copyright © Cassandra Farren 2019

ISBN: Paperback 978-0-9931296-8-1
ISBN: ebook 978-0-9931296-9-8

Front cover photograph © Donna Eade 2014
Front cover design © Fuzzy Flamingo
Author photograph © Kate Sharp Photography 2018
Editor Christine McPherson
A catalogue for this book is available from the

British Library.

*For Laura*
*Thank you for being there for me x*

# Introduction

"What's your name?" asked the woman sitting opposite me.

I stared at her in complete disbelief. Stunned into silence, I could feel a ripple of anger starting to build inside me. Pain spread across my chest, hurt ripped through my heart, as I fought back the burning tears in my eyes.

I wanted to shout, "How dare you ask me what my name is!" Instead, I blinked back my tears, forced a smile, and said, "My name is Cassie."

Her eyes softened, a gentle smile appeared on her face, and with all my might I prayed that she would remember.

Under normal circumstances, it would have been a seemingly innocent question. Two people meeting for the first time, intrigued to find out more about the person who had just entered their life.

But these were not normal circumstances. The woman opposite me was meant to love me, protect me, and be there for me, no matter what. It had been thirty-eight years since I first entered her life.

Why wasn't my name engraved on her soul?

The woman opposite me had given birth to me; she was the one who had chosen my name.

My world changed forever that day, with that simple but heart-breaking question. The question that should never have to be asked by any mother. The answer that should never have to be given by her child.

That was the moment when I knew.

I had lost my mum.

# Why am I writing this book?

I t's the 20<sup>th</sup> of November 2018. Today, is my second day of writing, and I am already seriously questioning myself. Have I got the emotional strength to finish what I've started? I set the intention that I would aim to write between 500 and 1000 words a day. Yesterday, I only managed 237 words before I had to stop, because I could no longer see the computer screen through my tears.

I love writing, but I already know that this book is going to challenge me on a whole new level. I have been told many times that I have *coped* surprisingly well over the last four years since my mum's diagnosis of dementia in November 2014. But I am human. I have moments when I sob over the awful injustice of watching the strong woman I once knew fade into a distant stranger I no longer recognise.

I am still experiencing the harrowing and lonely journey which has the potential to rip your world to pieces.

Having received very little support, I have had to find my own way. There have been countless times when I have felt afraid and scared.

I have held it together the best I can, because being strong is sometimes the only option. I am a single parent to my two boys; I may have lost my mum, but aged just sixteen and ten, they both still need theirs.

One of my philosophies in life is that you can give up or you can get up. I have managed to get up, time and time again, through many dark days and overcoming some huge life challenges.

You may feel by writing this book that I am a pretty tough cookie. But out of all the shit that life has dealt me, losing my mum to dementia is, hands-down, the hardest challenge I have ever had to face.

My mum was always a huge supporter of my work. She would always tell me how proud she was of my achievements. She loved that my business was making a difference to other people's lives. Mum would often say to me, "If you can do something that will help just one person, then I think you should do it."

So, *that* is why I am writing this book.

# Chapter One

*February 1, 2018*

"Sit down now! Look me in the eye and promise that you will never, ever, put me in a care home! I would rather die than be left in an institution. Tell me you would never do that. You are the only person I trust, Cassie. Swear on my life that you will never leave me there. Please, *please,* you have to promise me!"

I held back my tears, knowing that I was about to tell the biggest lie of my life to the woman I loved the most. Somehow, I looked her straight in the eye and replied, "I promise you, Mum, I will *never* do that."

*February 8, 2018*

That conversation I'd had with my mum just one week before was stuck in my head like a broken merry-go-round. I couldn't turn down the sound of the terror in my mum's voice. I couldn't get rid of the look of panic I had seen in her eyes; I couldn't erase the feeling of her gripping my hands tightly as she begged me to make a promise I knew I couldn't keep.

My day didn't start to plan, as my eldest son was in bed, too ill to go to school. At the age of 15, he was old enough to be left on his own, dosed up with medicine. I still felt bad about leaving him, but I didn't have time to wallow.

I got into my car and immediately turned up the music as loud as I could bear. I had driven to my parents' house hundreds of times before, but today was different. Today, I was making a heart-breaking journey that had the potential to haunt me for the rest of my life. As I started to drive, my head continued to spin. *Was this the right decision? Would my mum ever forgive me? And how on earth had it come to this?*

The music helped to drown out the questions, but it didn't stop a flood of memories replaying through my mind...

One morning in the summer of 2017, I had received a frantic call from my dad at 7.30am to say that my mum had gone missing and that the police had been called. She had gone downstairs to 'make a cup of tea' but had instead let herself out of the back gate and wandered off in nothing but her pyjamas and a pair of socks! Thankfully, she was found quickly at a friend's house.

Despite her being found safely, the whole incident had been extremely distressing. You hear on the news about people going missing, but you never think that it will happen to someone you love. We had known Mum was deteriorating, but we'd had no idea that she had become that bad. If you had met my mum at that point, it would not have been immediately apparent that she had dementia. She was a youthful-looking 69-year-old with lots of vibrancy and energy. Other than repeating herself, saying the odd random sentence and becoming more disorientated when she was out of her house, she still came across as fairly 'normal' to those who were unaware of her condition.

It had been two years since Mum's diagnosis, and in that time we hadn't received any support with the unforeseen challenges that come with caring for someone with dementia.

My mum had one appointment with her own doctor, who booked her in for some blood tests to rule out other conditions. He then referred her to the local memory clinic for some written and verbal tests.

The blood results were clear, and her low score from the memory clinic was confirmed. We received a letter to say Mum had dementia, along with prescribed medication to try and slow down the progression. There was a nurse who checked in on my mum for a few months to monitor any side-effects from the tablets… and that was it. We were then left to cope on our own.

Mum was in complete denial from day one and was convinced there was a conspiracy against her. Trying to get her to visit the doctor in the first place had been a complete nightmare. My dad asked her to go many times, but she would get angry and refuse because she insisted there was nothing wrong with her.

As time went on, I became increasingly concerned that her worsening symptoms might relate to something even more serious, like a brain tumour. I was explaining this on the phone to my dad one day, when my mum abruptly interrupted the conversation and said angrily, "Are you talking about me?" Unbeknown to us, Mum, who was starting to become paranoid, had picked up the other phone and had been listening to my concerns.

I had a split second to decide whether or not to make up an excuse, but I knew the situation needed to be dealt with. So, I took a deep breath and said, "Yes, Mum. We were talking about you. The reason is because we are really worried about you."

Ten minutes later, after lots of repeated questions from her and lots of repeated answers from me, I had somehow convinced her to visit her GP. In her mind, the visit was just to be on the safe side and to check that there was nothing wrong. In our minds, we suspected that there *was* something wrong and hoped that a medical diagnosis would be a step forward.

After the memory clinic diagnosis, Dad showed my mum the letter of confirmation from the doctor. But it only added to her conviction that even her doctor was in on the conspiracy against her!

Even though there were times when she knew *something* was wrong, Mum has never *believed* that she has dementia. When I arrived at her house on the morning she went missing, she was visibly upset and very angry.

She took me into the kitchen and said to me, "I don't understand, what is all the fuss about?"

I replied as calmly as I could, "Mum, you wandered off and were found at Sarah's house at 7.30am in your pyjamas."

Her response came in a raised voice. "Don't be so ridiculous! What on *earth* are you talking about? They are all against me, and I wish they would all f*ck off! Especially him upstairs (meaning my dad, who was on the phone to social services and cancelling the family holiday we were due to go on that morning). You can tell him to f*ck off as well!"

I had never heard my mum swear before, other than the very occasional bloody or bugger, but I'd certainly never heard her say the "F" word, and I'd never seen her in such a rage. How could I stop this?

My boys were only aged 8 and 14 at the time, so I had taken them with me to my parents' house that morning. I told Kieron, my eldest son, the truth about why we were no longer going away, but I bent the truth slightly with my youngest, Lennie, and said that Nana was poorly.

Mum's anger was still building as she walked out of the kitchen, and she pointed at Kieron and shouted, "Do *you* think I'm crazy, too?!"

At that point I wanted to scream, "ENOUGH!" No-one says the "F" word in front of my children, and no-one shouts at my children, especially when they've done nothing wrong. But what was I meant to do? I could hardly tell my mum off for swearing, as she would get even more upset and deny everything! I knew she genuinely had no recollection of what she'd said one minute before, let alone that she'd wandered off a few hours ago. It would be like me trying to convince you right now that you had been found wandering the streets in your pyjamas at 7.30am today. Of course you wouldn't believe me, and neither did my mum.

As I was desperately trying to distract and calm her down, Lennie put his hands over his ears and pleaded, "Please, will you all stop arguing?"

My heart was breaking. I felt physically and emotionally drained, and it was still only 10am. Mum was upset, my children were upset, and I was caught in the middle not knowing what to do for the best. We weren't having an argument as such, but as a family who never raises our voices this was not a nice atmosphere. Eventually, I managed to distract my mum from her angry questions and encouraged her to play in the garden with Lennie. I was then able to speak to my dad and discuss how to move forward, before we all had some lunch and pretended to my mum that nothing had happened.

I drove home at the end of a harrowing day, my mind in a daze. Now what? Where did we go from here? Dad had an alarm fitted on their front door, bought a large padlock for their back gate, and purchased a mobile tracker to locate Mum if she wandered off again. The police had also advised us to register my mum's details on their vulnerable person database. Up until this point I'd had no idea that such a thing even existed.

I remember feeling anxious as I opened a file of family photographs on my laptop. I hated the thought that whichever one I chose might one day be spread over the news and social media, should the worst happen.

I selected a photograph, and reminisced as I looked at the glint that had once been in my mum's eyes. She had grown up attending multiple schools, including some in Singapore and Malta, as her dad was in the Royal Air Force. Despite her education being, by her own admission, erratic at times, she succeeded in gaining her O levels and trained to become a teacher. And a very good teacher she was!

Mum loved her job and took her role to inspire and educate children very seriously. She cared about every single child she taught, not just the grades they gained. She would always get the job done, but as anyone who was taught by my mum would tell you, they had a lot of fun along the way! When she retired after 40 years of teaching, she used to volunteer weekly to hear the children read at the school where she used to teach.

Nothing was ever too much trouble, and she would always do whatever she could to help anyone. I remember her telling me about a time where she had been walking back from the town and saw an older lady who didn't look very well. Mum walked with her all the way to the health centre, got her some help, then phoned a taxi to take the woman back home!

When Kieron was born, like any grandchild he stole his grandparents' heart. I can still remember Mum meeting and holding him for the first time. She told me that she cried all the way home as the overwhelming love within her poured out. When Kieron didn't sleep at night, she would always offer to come and stay so that I could get some rest. If she visited at the weekend, Dad would drop her off, but at other times she thought nothing of walking to her local bus stop to catch her first bus, before waiting for a connection for her second bus, and then walk the rest of the way to my house. The entire journey would take two-and-a-half hours, and she would do the same trip in reverse to go home.

I'll never forget the devastating phone call I made to Mum when my first relationship ended. I can recall my mum answering in her positive and cheery voice, asking if I was okay. I can't remember the words that came out of my mouth, but I can vividly remember the most awful gut-wrenching feeling that I had let my parents down. They had done a fantastic job bringing up me and my sister; there had never been any pressure to bring home endless degrees or to pursue a certain career. All they wanted was for us to be happy. My voice quivered as I told my mum that something had happened which I couldn't accept. I told her that I had ended my relationship and was going to be living on my own with Kieron. She didn't inundate me with questions or try to tell me what to do. She was understandably shocked and upset, but her main concern was asking what could she do to help me. I was scared that if I couldn't keep my house, Kieron – only six months old at the time – and I could be re-housed in an area where we didn't feel safe. The upheaval of moving felt like too much to cope with on top of our lives unexpectedly collapsing.

I had only returned to work part-time some six weeks before the break-up, but I knew that I would need a full-time income in order to buy Kieron's dad out of the house. Kieron's nursery didn't have any full-time spaces for another six months, so I asked my mum if she could look after Kieron on the days when he wasn't at nursery. It meant that we could keep our house. Without hesitation, she said yes and we managed to fit the days around her teaching as she had reduced her hours to work part-time.

My mum was like a second mother to Kieron for the first few years of his life. As he and his little brother, Lennie – born six years later – grew up, she continued to love and cherish them both. There was nothing she loved more than spending time with her family and grandchildren.

# Chapter Two

Since they'd retired, my parents had spent several months at a time visiting my sister, Sam, and her family in New Zealand. Earlier in 2017, before Mum went missing, Dad had booked tickets to fly to New Zealand for what we knew would be one last time.

Understandably concerned after my mum's disappearance and not knowing whether to cancel the trip, Dad sought all the advice he could to ensure that my mum would be safe to travel. He phoned a dementia helpline and researched travelling abroad in the online help forums. He found many positive stories of hope and was encouraged to travel whilst they still could. We were also told by the doctor that Mum wandering off might have been a one-off occurrence due to a urine infection, which also gave him reassurance. So, after weighing up all the information and ensuring that my mum's tracker worked abroad, they set off on a journey that would never be forgotten.

★

My heart skipped a beat as a number from a foreign country flashed up on my mobile, I immediately feared the worst.

"Is that Cassie Farren?" asked a man with a stern accent.

"Yes, that's me."

"This is the duty manager. I've got your mother with me. She is extremely distressed, and she wants to speak to you."

What the hell had happened? Only a couple of hours earlier, I'd received a text from my dad to say they had landed in Singapore, where they would be spending four nights before flying on to New Zealand. He'd said the flight had gone well, and they had been out for some food. It would be the middle of the night there now.

The line went quiet before I heard my mum crying hysterically down the phone. She could hardly speak, but sobbed that 'they' were trying to drug her and that she didn't want to live any more. She said that she didn't want to see her family again, and told me to say goodbye to everyone she knew as she had had enough!

Sitting on my own several thousand miles away, listening to my mother breaking her heart, I felt so scared and helpless. Instinctively, I knew I had to calm her down and to keep her talking. So, I reassured her over and over again that she was safe and loved, whilst simultaneously praying for help. I don't know how long it took, but somehow, I managed to calm her down before the line went quiet again.

What was going on? There wasn't any point in asking my mum, as she clearly didn't know where she was. All I knew was that she was with the duty manager. But was he the duty manager of the police station? Had she been arrested? Was he the duty manager of the hospital? Was she ill? There was a small part of me that wanted to just hang up the phone, as it all felt too much. How was I meant to cope with this on my own?

When the duty manager came back on the phone, finally I managed to get some questions answered. He told me that my mum had woken up so confused and agitated that my dad had been concerned for her safety and called the duty manager of the hotel. I was relieved that she wasn't speaking to me from a police cell or hospital bed, but I knew the situation was still serious. The phone call to me, he said, had been made as a last resort because she had become too distressed and angry to be reasoned with.

The manager then explained that the hotel doctor was now with my mum, and had prescribed her a tablet to sedate and help her to sleep. He passed the phone to the doctor who assured me that Mum would be okay, but that she needed to sleep as soon as possible.

He said, "I am going to pass the phone back to your mum. She will be fine, but she really needs to sleep. You are the only one she trusts. Please tell her to take the tablet."

Could I really persuade her to take it? I took a deep breath, continued to pray, and then made up some nonsense that both her and my dad were going to take the tablet to help with jet lag. Whatever I said worked, thankfully, as she gradually became more relaxed. The line then went quiet again before Dad came on the phone and said that she'd taken the tablet.

Naturally, my dad was extremely upset by what had happened. Despite the doctor assuring him that Mum would be fine after some sleep, he felt that flying to New Zealand was going to be too much for both of them. We agreed that he should try and get some rest and make a final decision in the morning, but that I would call my sister and tell her that there was a good chance they wouldn't be visiting her now.

11

I ended the call and took a moment to try and take in what had just happened, before phoning my sister. Instead of meeting our parents from the airport in a few days' time, I had to tell her it was more likely they'd be on a flight back to England.

The next morning, Dad confirmed that he wanted to come home, so I agreed to rearrange their flights. The travel agent I spoke to was extremely understanding, despite my dad having to pay some extra money it was a relatively straight forward process. They were scheduled to land into Heathrow Airport late on Friday afternoon. I just wanted to get the text to say they'd landed safely so we could all put this nightmare behind us.

That afternoon, I got the text I'd been waiting for. But the nightmare was far from over.

# Chapter Three

TEXT FROM DAD: *Just landed. Mum collapsed when she got off the plane. Waiting for an ambulance. Battery very low will update you as soon as I can.*

Mum has collapsed? Needs an ambulance? What does that mean? Was she unconscious? Alive? It was the longest 45 minutes of my life as I stared helplessly at my mobile phone and waited. I didn't want to use my phone in case Dad was trying to call. I knew my sister was waiting for an update to say they'd arrived safely, but there was no point in worrying her until I knew more information. I didn't know what to do. So, I paced the house and prayed.

I nearly cried with relief when Dad eventually called and I could hear my mum talking in the background. She was alive! He explained that the doctors thought she might have a blood clot, but they'd done some initial tests and the situation wasn't urgent. They were now waiting for a scan, as a precaution, but it could be a few hours before they knew for sure. It was now 10pm, so Dad told me to rest and that he'd text once they had the results. I spoke briefly to my mum, who sounded upbeat and reassured me that the doctors were looking after her. Thank God for that!

When we ended the call, I updated my sister, who had

already made the decision to catch the next flight back to England so she could support my parents for ten days once they arrived home. Then I went to bed, feeling shaken up but relieved that Mum was going to be okay.

When my phone rang at 11pm, I expected to hear that they'd got the scan results and that everything was alright. I wasn't expecting to be on my way to London 15 minutes later. The scan had identified multiple, large blood clots. According to the doctor, Mum's condition was life-threatening.

Thankfully, Lennie was staying with his dad and my next-door neighbour was able to stay at my house to look after Kieron. I prayed all the way to London, not knowing if she was dead or alive and when I arrived at the Intensive Care Unit, I feared the worst when the nurse told me that my mum wasn't there. Was I too late? I called Dad, who confirmed she was in the Coronary Care Unit. In the panic of the initial phone call, I had misheard the abbreviation of CCU and thought she was in ICU!

By the time I arrived at the correct ward, I already felt emotionally drained. Mum didn't look well, but she was conscious. The doctors explained that all they could do was to give her six months' worth of blood-thinning drugs intravenously over the next 48 hours. In no uncertain terms, we were told that there would be one of two outcomes: the drip would dissolve the clots and my mum would live; or the drip would not dissolve the clots, they would travel to her heart and she would die.

I didn't have time to process the severity of this information as Mum had decided she wanted to go home and was attempting to rip the life-saving drip out of her arm! She was scared, afraid, and in pain, but her behaviour was becoming aggressive. She had no idea where she was and was adamant that she wanted to get off her bed, but she was still attached to the drip which was saving her life.

The staff were fantastic in providing her medical care, but it shocked me that none of them could speak to Mum in a way she understood. They kept on repeating to her, "You're in hospital. You are extremely ill. You need to stay on your bed." All this did was add to her frustration, and she became increasingly angry. She began to scream, shout, and swear, whilst still trying to rip the drip out of her arm. If she succeeded in her mission, there was a good chance that she would bleed to death because her blood was so thin.

I kept trying to calm my mum down, but it was impossible. It was late, and the staff were not happy as she was causing a commotion and disturbing the other patients. I begged them to try and sedate her, but there was only so much medication they could give in case it had a negative effect on the blood-thinning drugs. Every minute felt like an hour, and at one point there was me and four members of staff restraining her as she continued to scream, swear, and cry. *This is not my mum!* I kept thinking. *Where is my mum? Please can someone bring back my mum!*

For the rest of the night, I sat on a plastic chair, bending over the metal rail on my mum's bed, holding her down whilst trying to comfort, calm, and reassure her that she wasn't being attacked or burgled.

I prayed all night for a miracle, and it came in the form of a new doctor who immediately took control of the situation. He spoke to my mum in a much more compassionate way and even had her smiling.

When her breakfast arrived, she was so weak that I had to cut the food up and feed it to her. It felt so wrong. Even one month earlier Mum would have told me that she didn't need any help with *anything,* thank you very much. That strong woman had faded away so quickly, it scared me that she could slip away at any given moment. But there was nothing we could do except pray that the clots were dissolving.

The next 48 hours were very touch-and-go. Mum was calmer and co-operating, but it was awful knowing that everything could change in the blink of an eye. We were told by the doctor that they couldn't transfer her to a hospital closer to home, as there was a good chance she might not survive the journey. And until they performed the next scan in 24 hours' time, it was still a life or death situation which could go either way.

My next-door neighbour and Lennie's dad had been helping so that I could stay at the hospital, but on the second night I didn't have any childcare, so I had to go home. I nearly cried as I hugged her and said goodbye, not knowing if I would see her alive again. She looked me in the eyes and said, "I'll see you again soon. I love you, Sunshine" – the name she'd often call me. I managed to hold it together, until I walked out of the ward.

Back home, I hardly slept all night as I was constantly checking my phone. Thankfully, the call I was dreading never came, and I headed back to the hospital on the Sunday morning. The doctors were pleased with Mum's progress but kept reminding us that they wouldn't know if the blood clots had dissolved until they carried out the scan the next day.

My sister arrived at the hospital on Sunday afternoon, which cheered my mum up no end. She kept telling the doctors how happy she was to have all of her family with her.

I went home again that evening feeling calmer, but still worried about the outcome of the scan. *What if the blood clots hadn't dissolved and there was nothing more they could do?* Once again, I prayed for a miracle.

My stomach sank when I saw my dad's number flash up on my phone the following morning. But he told me that a miracle had happened! Mum had been for her scan, and the blood clots had all completely disappeared! I had no idea if this was due to the drugs, the prayers, or a combination of both, but in that moment I didn't care.

It felt like we had been given some extra time with my mum, who was very happy that she could finally leave the hospital. She was discharged later that day with three months' worth of blood-thinning tablets and a check-up booked at her local hospital in six weeks' time.

It just goes to show how quickly your life can change. On the Friday afternoon my mum had been rushed into hospital with life-threatening blood clots, yet on the Monday afternoon she was on her way home, none the wiser. That's right, she had no idea. Thankfully, her dementia had completely wiped any recollection of her hospital visit.

Unfortunately, the same couldn't be said for me. I tried to block out that awful first night, but my mind replayed it over and over again. I could still hear the heart-wrenching sound of my mum screaming as I relived how helpless I had felt. For the next three weeks, I was ill – possibly caused by stress.

I'll be honest. Before my mum was taken into hospital, I had found myself becoming increasingly frustrated with her. In the good old days, we always used to have a laugh and a giggle. But as her condition progressed, she became paranoid and angry, and it became harder to have a conversation with her, or with anyone else in the same room.

My mum and dad had often driven over to my house to visit me and the boys. I used to open the door to my 'old' mum, who would exclaim, "Cassie! It's so good to see you, let me give you a hug!" She would immediately want to know how I was, how the boys were, and what we had all been up to.

But more recently, I would open the door to my 'new' mum, who would stand on my doorstep looking like a sad, lost child, often with tears in her eyes. I would have to coax her to come into my house, where she would either quietly sulk and not say a word, or mutter in an angry tone, "I don't know why I'm here. Nobody told me I was coming, and don't you dare let *him* leave me here!" My dad would walk in behind her, looking upset, saying that he had told her all morning and all the way here where she was going.

Of course I wanted to spend time with my mum, but it felt more and more like hard work. She began to understand less, which meant she couldn't join in with a 'normal' conversation. If Dad tried to speak to me about anything, she would either sit in silence looking upset or talk over us, repeating one of her childhood stories. Even simple questions like, "Would you like a cup of tea?" became a challenge. She'd say no, then I'd make a cup for myself and she'd get in a mood and say that she wanted one. Or she'd say, yes, then forget she'd said yes and would be confused why I had made her one. I know that may sound like a tiny problem, but when you have to handle these challenges one after the other for four or five hours, it didn't feel like the quality family time we'd once shared.

Dad was becoming increasingly tired, and I always felt bad when they left to go home. I would be upset that another week had passed and I'd lost another part of my mum, but felt worse that my dad had no break and had to drive home and deal with these challenges day in, day out, on his own.

# Chapter Four

After Mum's miraculous recovery in hospital, it seemed like she'd been given a second chance and I felt blessed that I had more time to spend with her, even if that meant adapting to the 'new' mum who was increasingly forgetting who I was.

It was as though she was lost in between two worlds; she was neither here nor there. As an example, when my mum would visit, she would reluctantly come into my house in the way I described earlier. I would then endeavour to calm her down and offer her a cup of tea, which as you now know wasn't straightforward. We would then have about two sentences of normal conversation of, "How have you been?" before she'd throw something randomly into the conversation like, "Well, I never agreed with the man from the town who wanted to buy a sofa from the dog who used to visit me when I was teaching before my friend's auntie went to the supermarket."

I quickly learned that if I corrected her or said, "I'm not sure what you mean", she would immediately snap back into sulking mode or silently stare into space.

I discovered that if I found a way to carry on the conversation in a normal tone by saying, "Oh right, that sounds interesting" then she could confidently carry on the conversation with something else like, "So I told the doctor the yellow flowers faded after I saw the horse at the school before we went back to the coffee shop." It was incredibly hard at first to keep the conversation going, but the more I tried hard to make an effort with my answers, the more she would continue to speak.

I also noticed that a huge part of her reaction depended on my body language and the emotion behind my words. Talking to Mum required full-on concentration, because I never knew what she was going to say at any given moment. But I knew that if I could look interested, smile, and find a way to carry on speaking with positivity, then her anxiety vastly decreased. I believe this was because she no longer felt like she was being considered to be stupid, which was something she was paranoid about.

I can't imagine how it must feel to be trapped in a brain that is fading away. She'd say things like, "I know I must have told you this one hundred times before, and I'm sure you think I'm really thick." I would reassure her that she hadn't told me before (even though she'd just told me four times in a row!) and that I didn't think she was thick, but she'd instantly forget and then ask me again.

When I learned that my emotions had a direct impact on hers, I began to mentally prepare myself for her visits. I'm aware this may sound strange, but it really worked. When my parents were due to visit, I would endeavour to stop working 30 minutes before their arrival. I would sit quietly and listen to some relaxing music or do some meditation, so that when they arrived, I had cleared my own emotions (even if only temporarily) to leave me in the best possible state to help to manage my mum's emotions.

I would still answer the door to a sullen-looking mum, who was still angry, upset, and anxious. But instead of me thinking, 'Here we go again' and feeling tense, I intentionally started to put up an invisible glass wall between myself and my emotions so that I could give all of my positivity and attention to her.

I would take a deep breath, open the door with a big smile, and immediately give her a compliment like, "Hi Mum, I love your jumper, that blue looks great on you. Come on in. I want to show you the flowers that have come up in the garden. I was wondering if you could help me in the garden today?" Then I'd lead her through the kitchen, open the back door, walk outside, and give her another compliment like, "It made such a difference when you picked those leaves up last time. Would you be able to help me pick up some more today?"

By this point, she would have calmed down, and more often than not I would even get a smile. She would still say something like, "I'm sorry to get upset. I just didn't know where we were going today." But I would deflect the conversation back to her helping me. "Oh well, never mind, I'm happy that you're here now. If you can help me with these leaves, that would be great. I'll get a bag."

I had also learned that she wanted to feel useful. Asking her to complete a task that she could do, like picking up leaves, made her very happy. I could then come back inside and say, 'Hi Dad, how are you?' and we'd have a catch-up once my mum was settled.

When I changed my emotional state, made Mum the

priority in the initial conversation, stopped correcting her, tried to carry on any conversation she started, and gave her manageable tasks, she was much less anxious and our time together felt so much better. At the end of every visit, Mum would always spring back in to 'old mum' mode by giving hugs and high-fives to me and the boys. She'd tell me that I was an amazing mum and how proud she was of me.

I always felt tired and emotional after they left, as it took a lot of effort and concentration to manage the situation. But at least I had the opportunity to rest and get a good night's sleep once they'd gone. Unfortunately, the same couldn't be said for my dad, and he was increasingly feeling the strain of changing roles from being Mum's husband to becoming her full-time carer.

Thirty-eight years ago he had married a woman who was always confident, independent, and full of life. Now, she was often angry, confused and anxious, and to make things worse she didn't recognise him a lot of the time. On top of his emotional exhaustion, there was the physical fatigue. My dad did whatever he could to support Mum, but the fact remained that he had not had a proper break or a decent night's sleep for months.

I tried to support Dad as much as I could, but I was also running a business, working freelance around school hours, writing my second book, and bringing up my children. I'd had a difficult few years since my life had collapsed for the third time in 2016. I had picked up the pieces and come so far emotionally, but I was still trying to get back on track financially.

The obvious answer to increase financial stability would be to get a full-time job. But this would mean accepting the many challenges of working around school hours and holidays, not to mention if one of the boys was ill. I had worked in full-time and part-time employment for many years when the boys were younger, but I no longer had the back up of my mum's extra support if I needed it. It would also mean I couldn't continue to give my dad a break, if I was to go down this road.

Despite losing so much I still I believed in myself and in my business. So I did what I always did. I worked hard, juggled my responsibilities, and carried on in the hope that all my work would eventually pay off.

I would endeavour to see my parents at least one day each week and every other weekend. In that time, I would take Mum in the garden for a few hours or out for a long walk to give her some exercise whilst my dad had some time to sleep. It was hard to see him looking so tired. And even though visiting us gave him a little respite, it had reached the point where he needed more.

Not only could he not leave my mum on her own any more, but he couldn't even make any phone calls while she was in the house. She had become more paranoid, especially if she thought that anyone was speaking about her. She was still convinced that there was nothing wrong with her, and that we were all ganging up against her. So, from then on, I took charge when it came to making telephone calls.

# Chapter Five

I decided to call one of the nurses at the memory clinic to ask for some advice on how my dad could receive some more support. She told me, "Your mum does not have capacity; she is dangerous because she looks so young and disguises her condition so well. She needs professional care and to be out walking every day to lessen the chance that she will wander off again."

It was hard to hear my mum being described in this way, but I knew that the nurse was being honest, and she didn't want my mum to come to any harm. She advised that we should have a carer twice a week to take Mum out, which would give my dad some much-needed rest.

Part of me didn't want to tell Dad this information. I didn't want him thinking that we didn't believe he was capable of looking after my mum, but by his own admission, he was exhausted. After a few very honest conversations, he agreed that I should start making some enquiries with local care agencies.

I wasn't sure what to expect, but surely it couldn't be hard to arrange care for four hours a week? It wasn't as though Mum needed any physical care like getting dressed, or anything. We just needed someone who would be like a professional friend. Someone who would understand her needs and take her out for a walk, or on a visit to a garden centre.

After hours of trying to find a suitable agency, I was running out of hope. Suddenly, I remembered about a care agency where I had been offered a job a few years before. Yes, you read that right. For a period when my business wasn't doing well, I took a job as a carer and underwent all of the training. I didn't end up accepting the position, but I remembered that this particular company offered companionship care. I called them and was very relieved to find out that they did have some availability. I was advised to get the ball rolling quickly, as it could take several weeks to get everything set up, so we booked an initial telephone consultation for the next day.

I had to relay the information to my dad in e-mails, as we couldn't have any conversations without Mum getting cross. We agreed there wasn't any way of telling her that she would be having carers, as she would definitely not accept them. Yes, her dementia was getting worse, but she still had a very strong sense of 'knowing.' There had been several occasions when people had visited the house to check her medication which had distressed her, and she was becoming increasingly suspicious with any new people. If she was left with me whilst my dad went out for a few hours, she would become really stressed and ask me, "Where's he gone? When's he coming back? Has he gone to book me into a care home?" And these same questions would be asked on repeat until Dad returned.

I kept reminding myself that, despite our concerns, we had to put Mum's safety before our emotions. The nurse

I had spoken to had categorically told me that I needed to arrange this care, along with respite for my dad, and she wanted an update from me in one month's time. I knew she was concerned, and so was I. It would be much better to make plans now than to face an emergency situation which resulted in Mum being taken into a care home, or worse, being sectioned if she was deemed to be a risk to herself. I had read on several online help forums about this happening when people went missing, and it was one of my worst nightmares.

It felt so surreal having the telephone consultation and answering questions about my mum's needs, it was as though we were speaking about someone else. To my relief, they told me that their staff didn't wear uniforms. That had been one of our concerns, as we didn't want Mum to suspect they were carers. The only worry was that they needed to send forms for my dad to sign, and to carry out two assessments – one of which had to be conducted at my parents' house. I reassured Dad that we had to trust that everything would work out okay, and simply handle one step at a time.

Mum was paranoid about letters, especially anything which looked medical. Thankfully we already had the health and financial Power of Attorney's in place. These are documents that enable someone to appoint 'attorneys', a trusted friend and/ or relative, to manage their health and financial matters. The care agency agreed that my dad could sign all of the forms and that they would send the letters in his name only. They also agreed that I could attend the initial assessment on my own, and text Dad if there were any questions I couldn't answer.

We scheduled all of the arrangements and assessments to take place during the school holidays, though I was already juggling a lot with the boys. I ended the phone call to the agency feeling so guilty for 'betraying' my mum, who had always begged us never to arrange any kind of care. I also felt apprehensive knowing how my dad felt about bending the truth, as he would face the repercussions from my mum if everything went belly-up.

I ended the call and could have done with a power nap, but I had just ten minutes to make the boys some lunch before a business adviser was phoning me. I had found out about some local business funding which I was eligible for, and I was hoping it could give my business a much-needed boost. They were awarding grants and support to businesses in the area who wanted to grow and expand. I had been told that an adviser was going to go through a business analysis, which was the first stage of the funding application. I gave myself a quick talking to and reminded myself that this was a positive opportunity and that it would give me something to focus on. How wrong could I have been?

I had a quick lunch, answered the call, and for the next hour I was grilled by one of the most negative and condescending people I have ever spoken to. He asked me, "Why do you think your business hasn't been successful? Why aren't you making more profit? Do you really believe you have what it takes to make this work?" As the inquisition went on, my positivity and self-belief vanished. Have you ever had a conversation with someone where, in hindsight, you wished you had stuck up for yourself and given them a piece of your mind?

I wanted to say, "Have you read my book, *The Girl Who*

*Refused to Quit?* Have you got any idea what I have been through to get to this point?" He had no idea that I had still been hopeful of success, despite my heart breaking over Mum's condition, and trying to do my best running a business as a single parent, but his infectious negativity made me question everything. Maybe he was right. Maybe I didn't have what it takes. Maybe I should just quit.

In that moment, I didn't have any more to give. I tried to explain that I did consider my business to be successful and that I had already changed many people's lives. No, I wasn't making a huge profit, but neither were many large companies in this country! It's not easy to make a profit when you invest everything you earn back into your business. I explained that I had set up my business as a single parent with nothing more than a Facebook page, and that I'd had to learn everything myself from scratch, which takes hard work, time and dedication. I shared how becoming a single parent for the third time just one year ago, after a new relationship had collapsed, had also impacted my business. I had found a way to carry on despite having to move to a new house and start life again with my children. Not only had I been running my business and working freelance I had also written another book in only two months!

I explained that once my new book was published, I would be running workshops, online programmes, and intended to increase my work as a speaker.

However, I could tell from his tone that it was unlikely he believed in me. He confirmed this by saying that, despite running my business for over four years, he would put me into the 'start-up' category, and the forms would be e-mailed to me that afternoon.

I hung up the phone and burst into tears. I was angry with the adviser, but I was also upset with myself. His question continued to spin around in my head, "Do you really believe you've got what it takes to make this work?" As I sat sobbing in my kitchen, the honest answer was no, I didn't. I had worked so hard to inspire people despite my own life being turned upside down again, but I couldn't do this on my own any more. Where was my support? Why wouldn't anyone give me a chance?

# Chapter Six

A few days later, I was sitting in my parents' living room. My mum was upstairs, so my dad took the five-minute window of opportunity to speak to me about my business before Mum came back and we would have to revert to the basic conversations she could understand.

"How did the application for your funding go?" he asked.

I tried to inject some positivity into my voice and began to say, "Not as well as I had hoped..." But then my voice cracked, and the involuntary tears began to fall. I repeated the negative feedback I had received as quickly as I could, whilst watching the sadness build in my dad's eyes as his normally strong daughter spoke like a vulnerable child.

Just then, I heard Mum walking down the stairs, so I had to abruptly end the conversation and wipe away my tears. I dried my eyes and had to accept there would be no more talking about the support I needed, as my mum would either ask me the same question a million times over or she would sit and sulk that she couldn't join in the conversation. Either way, there was a chance I might snap at her after the week I'd had. Yes, she had dementia. Yes, I loved her. And yes, I put her needs first. But right then, I needed my mum – and once again, she couldn't be there for me.

It was like *déjà vu* as I remembered being sat in exactly the same chair having exactly the same thought only one year before.

★

When my new relationship abruptly ended in 2016, to say the shit hit the fan would be an understatement. There is *nothing* that can prepare you for becoming a single parent for the third time. Once is hard; twice is devastating; three times…well, it just shouldn't happen.

One of my challenges was to find a new house and move in as quickly as we could. If you've ever moved to a new house, you will know that this is a very stressful time under normal circumstances. But in my case, this was anything but normal, and would have been more suited to a month-long special of a television drama! I'm not sure how I coped with the ridiculous amount of pressure of having our lives torn apart for the third time.

My nerves were already hanging by a thread as I packed up our belongings, worked twelve hours a day on a new online programme, and tried to support the boys. Everything was planned and I was counting down the days until we moved out. Then I received an unexpected call from my landlord to say that there was a problem with the boiler in the new house. It wouldn't be fixed until the following Wednesday, so he would need to postpone our moving-in date by four days. Four days doesn't sound like a big deal, except that: a) I didn't want to stay in that house a minute longer than we had to; and b) my ex-partner was returning to the house on the Saturday, so there was no way that we were going to still be there.

The boxes were packed, the removal men were booked for the Saturday, and everything was set to be launched for my programme on the Monday. What the hell was I going to do? Part of me wanted to drink a bottle of wine and give up on being an adult for a while. Why did it have to be so bloody hard? After a few tears of frustration (and a small glass of wine!), I decided that we *would* be moving out on Saturday and my programme *would* be launched on Monday. I would find a way.

Let's be honest, there aren't many people who find it easy to ask for help. Society has conditioned us to keep calm and carry on, because we are all invincible and we can cope with anything, can't we? But this wasn't a time to be proud. I needed support, and time wasn't on my side. So, I swallowed my pride and asked for help. I arranged for the boys to stay with their dads, I went to stay at my parents' house, and I moved our furniture to our new house on the Saturday as planned.

On the moving day, I felt exhausted driving to my mum and dad's house. I was trying to process how a few short weeks before, I'd had what I thought was a settled life, and now I was going to be without a home for four nights. It goes without saying that I was grateful to have a roof over my head, as I've volunteered for a homeless charity and will never take for granted what I do have in my life. But I felt so empty. I just wanted to move into our new house so that we could start to rebuild our life again.

When I arrived, Mum asked if I'd like a cup of tea. Honestly? A bottle of wine would have been my preference, but to be fair, it was only 11.30am! I told her that I would love one, thank you. Two hours passed, and I had been asked over 20 times if I would like a cup of tea, but the tea never appeared. Mum would go into the kitchen to make the tea before forgetting what she was there for and walk back out of the kitchen. Five minutes later, she would repeat the same process.

I tried to resolve the situation by offering her a cup of tea, but she would insist that she was perfectly capable of making a cup of tea… and then she'd forget again. On a 'normal' day, this was 'normal' behaviour – no cup of tea, no problem. But that day, I remember thinking, I just wanted a cup of tea and a chat with my mum. Was that too much to ask? Instead, she kept asking me over and over again how my ex-partner was. Was he at work? Was he coming over later? Where were the boys? What time was I collecting them from school? And still no cup of tea.

In between these questions, she would repeat her favourite childhood stories over and over again. Still no cup of tea. Every time my dad left the room, I would then be forced to listen to her slating him and telling me, "He thinks I'm mad. Did you know he won't let me out of the house on my own?" She'd then ask me, "Do you think I'm mad? Do you think I'm demented?" I managed to deflect all of these questions to then be faced with the question I dreaded the most: "Where's my mum? Is she dead?" Her own mum and dad had both passed away many years before.

If you've never heard the phrase 'love lies' before, these are lies that are told to avoid hurting or upsetting the person with dementia. So, I tried with all my might to answer her questions with a calm voice and tell as many 'love lies' as I needed to, but in all honesty, I just wanted a hug and a bloody cup of tea.

★

I snapped myself out of the temporary daydream I had fallen into, and back into the present moment. Mum had now decided to go out and pick up some leaves in the garden, so I quickly got my diary out and told Dad about the plans to get the companionship care in place. They needed to come to my parents' house to do an initial assessment on my mum. I knew my dad wasn't keen on this – neither was I, to be fair – but there was no other way. They needed to ask Mum some questions and to check the house as part of their setting-up procedures.

They had assigned my mum two carers, who would need to come to the house separately to be introduced to her. Dad and I were both still very apprehensive about this as Mum's suspicion of strangers always strengthened her conviction that we were conspiring against her. She was still adamant that there was nothing wrong with her, but we knew she was getting worse. There had been a recent episode of her wandering off when Dad went upstairs for five minutes, innocently assuming that she was safely downstairs. He'd then received a phone call to say she had turned up at her friend's house, distraught that Dad had gone out and left her! We needed to put our apprehension to one side and remind ourselves that her safety had to come first.

To try and ease Mum's suspicions, I suggested that I would drive to her house, meet each carer outside, and we would go into the house together where I would introduce the carer as my friend. I would tell a love lie that my friend had moved into the area and wanted to meet some new people. I felt guilty and apprehensive breaking my mum's trust, but it had to be done. Either the hard work would pay off and Dad would get some much-needed rest, or the shit would hit the fan and all hell would break loose. We would soon find out.

# Chapter Seven

*20<sup>th</sup> August, 2017*

From: Sam
To: Dad and Cassie
*Just wanted to say hope all goes well tomorrow... I'll be thinking of you all. xxxx*

*21<sup>st</sup> August, 2017*

From: Cassie
To: Sam
*Thanks, Sam – I've got no idea what to expect, to be honest, but praying it all goes ok.*

*Mum wasn't too good yesterday as she told dad her tooth really hurt – he took her to the out-of-hours dentist but then she got upset as she didn't know why she was there. She has an infection in her tooth, so she was given antibiotics, but then she didn't understand why she had to take them and was cross she had to take another tablet, etc.*

*They came here and Dad slept for 2 hours; he's not been very well. He said he's been sweating and shivering over the last few days.*

*Me and Mum did some gardening and went for a walk so Dad could have a break. I really hope today goes ok. I'll let you know. xx*

## 21st August, 2017

From: Cassie
To: Dad and Sam

*I feel like it went really well today. I walked into the house with the two ladies – supervisor Anne and carer Michelle. Me, Mum, and Michelle went in the garden whilst Dad and Anne chatted and did a risk assessment.*

*We then came back inside and had a cup of tea, and they were encouraging Mum to speak about the good old days. I don't think Mum suspected anything, and was chatting and laughing and seemed to really enjoy their company. When they went, they both said they thought it went well so all in all a very good first step.*

*I will be going back on Thursday when it's Michelle's first official day. I will then go back over again next Tuesday when it's the other carer Tia's first day.*

*Cassie x*

## 29th August, 2017

From: Cassie
To: Dad and Sam

*I thought it went well again today, Mum chatted very happily to Tia about her past.*

See you Thursday. If you remind Mum that my friend is coming round, before Michelle arrives on her own. Fingers crossed it will go ok.

Cassie x

30th August, 2017

To: Cassie and Sam
From: Dad
*Hi Cassie & Sam,*

*Mum was a bit confused after Tia had gone. Strangely asking if I had written up the visit? During the evening Mum asked many times where her mum and dad had gone, and at bedtime she kept asking all sorts of questions relating to our family.*

*All my love,*
*Dad*

30th August, 2017

To: Cassie and Dad
From: Sam
*Hi Dad and Cass,*

*Sorry to hear Mum got a little confused yesterday. I imagine it may just be due to a few new things going on. Hope today is better. Sounds like Mum has been accepting of the new carers. Are they nice people? What have they been doing with Mum? Just hanging out at home or have they been walking, etc?*

*Catch up soon. xxx*

*30ᵗʰ August, 2017*

To: Dad and Sam
From: Cassie

*They've both done one session each and wanted to get to know Mum, so they chatted at home both times and had a cup of tea. They are both very good at active listening, e.g. letting Mum talk about whatever she wants to talk about, they don't interrupt, correct her, or talk about themselves that much. They just listen and agree with whatever Mum says, which makes her happy and boosts her confidence as she feels like she is in control. She's been happy both times. Tomorrow will be the first time Mum will be on her own with Michelle, as I won't be there.*

*Cassie x*

*1ˢᵗ September, 2017*

To: Cassie and Sam
From: Dad
*Hi Sam & Cassie,*

*Yesterday started well. Michelle arrived, and I made a cup of tea. Mum was chatting away with her for fifteen minutes before I said I was just popping up to B&Q. I got home two hours later, and they were still chatting.*

*Before Michelle left she said that Mum kept on asking her who she was, why was she there, and who does she work for!? Also, Mum said to me, "Is Michelle writing a report on me?"*

*After Michelle left, Mum asked me the same questions*

*again before and during our journey over to your house, Cassie.*

*During our meal together, Mum was very distant. It could have been the loud music, she was confused due to many things going on, or was over-tired?*

*It didn't get any better when we got home. Mum just sat in the chair with her arms crossed tightly, not talking. Eventually, after just gently rubbing the back of her hand, she slowly started to talk and cry. She wanted to know where her dad was and said that he was here an hour ago! I used all my usual techniques and eventually calmed Mum down and went to bed at 10.30pm.*

*This morning we woke about 7am. Mum was asking her usual questions, then after about forty-five minutes she went to sleep and didn't get up again until 12.45pm! So, it may have been that she was very tired yesterday? (It was about 2.30am the previous night before Mum went to sleep, after about two hours of answering her questions!)*

*This is just a quick resume of what happened, we will have to see how the next few visits work out.*

*All my love,*
*Dad*

*5th September, 2017*

To: Dad and Sam
From: Cassie
*Hi Dad and Sam,*

*I spoke to the care company this morning who were very understanding of our concerns that Mum was a bit* upset last week. I asked if Mum could start going out and about on the visits. I have only spoken to Dad on text, but he said it went much better and they went to the park and had a cup of tea. He said that Mum did ask who Tia was, but Dad has been answering and saying that she's my friend.

I'm feeling a lot better than I was, although I've been really tired and falling asleep in the afternoons. I will have to make today the last day of that as both boys go back to school tomorrow so need to get fully back in work mode.

In other news, I've had the final copy of my book cover back today. I'm really happy with it!

Cassie x


6th *September, 2017*

From: Cassie
To: Dad and Sam

*Just to throw a spanner in the works, the care company called today and said that Tia is struggling to keep up with mum's pace when they go out walking. They are going to replace her with a new carer called Claire, starting from Tuesday.*

*I thought they would have taken this into consideration before matching her with Mum but didn't see the point in starting a conflict as it won't change anything. I did say that I hope it doesn't cause too much confusion for Mum as she is only just getting used to them. They just suggested that I go over again and introduce her as my friend to ease the blow.*

*Dad: I will come over on Tuesday at 1pm to meet Claire. I will only be able to stay for forty-five minutes as need to collect Lennie from school and drop him at his swimming lesson before I drive to an evening meeting in Peterborough.*

*I'll see you on Friday.*

*Cassie x*

# Chapter Eight

*September 2017*

While we were adjusting to the new carers, I had started to research into care homes which could potentially provide a couple of nights' respite for my dad. The new companionship care had brought some temporary relief, but what he really longed for most was a decent sleep. He was relieved that he could now go food shopping, or pop out and get a paper without the ordeal of getting my mum ready and out of the house. I say ordeal as it could take up to two hours to get my mum to *agree* to get ready and leave home. She might put a summer dress on in the winter and insist that's what she was wearing; she could burst out crying for no reason, or insist that she packed and re-checked her bag fifty times before leaving the house. And it was not unusual for her to ask my dad over and again where they were going, why they were going, and who they were meeting, and then decide, having gone through all of this, that she wasn't going anywhere.

At the end of every long day, having dealt with the many challenges of being a full-time carer, you would think that sitting down with a coffee to relax in front of the TV would be in order. In reality, that's when the real challenges started.

Many dementia patients become increasingly anxious and agitated in the evenings. There were many occasions when my mum would hallucinate, get upset, and decide that she wanted to get out of the house. If Dad managed to calm her down, his next hurdle was to convince Mum to take her medication. If this was managed, the next task was to get her to go to bed.

There were many evenings when Mum wouldn't go to bed until the early hours of the morning. And due to her increasing confusion, she would often think my dad was someone else, tell him to get out of her bed, then pace around the house or quiz him with multiple questions before she would finally fall asleep. In Dad's case, he was often too anxious to sleep and was constantly just napping before starting what felt like Groundhog Day the next morning. Friends were kind enough to look after my mum for a few hours, and I helped as much as I could, but this pattern was becoming Dad's life, day in day out, and he needed a proper break.

It was really difficult to bring myself to start researching care homes. Even though I was only looking into respite care at that stage, we all knew what this meant longer-term as my mum continued to decline. She was still so young; how could this be fair? Fair or not, no-one else was going to make those dreaded phone calls.


*18th October, 2017*

To: Dad and Sam
From: Cassie

*Hi Dad and Sam,*

*Just to update you, Sam, me and Dad had a chat when he came over, and Dad doesn't feel booking extra time with the carers will help. Dad would really like to have a whole night – or two – when he can properly rest and relax and recharge.*

*I've just spoken to a care home which has some space, and have arranged a visit for Tuesday 24th at 2.15pm. Dad, can you meet me there?*

*I said the main problem is that Mum has absolutely no idea that she has dementia, and would completely freak out at being told she was going to stay at a care home, so we would need to lie and perhaps say Dad was going into hospital, or anything else we can think of?*

*She said not to worry for now, to come and have a look around and ask any questions, then go from there. She said they are used to managing people, and that the majority of people there think they are in a hotel and it doesn't feel like a care home.*

*Cassie x*

I had been as positive as I could on the drive to visit the first care home. I reminded myself that my dad desperately needed a break and that Mum would be safe and well looked after. I had to trust that this was the next step on our journey and told myself that my mum would be okay.

Having not been into a care home for twenty years since my nan passed away, I wasn't sure what to expect, but it certainly wasn't this. As soon as I walked in, I felt uneasy. We had to wait for ten minutes as they were running late due to staff shortages; not a great first impression. We were then given a rushed tour through the dark, twisting corridors that made me feel claustrophobic and confused! How on earth would my mum cope? We were then told that not every room had an en-suite, and my mum would be given whatever room was available on the day. How would my mum find the toilet and her way back to the room at night in a strange environment?

As we made our way around the day lounges, I started to feel like I wanted to leave. It became apparent why I had heard people refer to some care homes as 'God's waiting room', as everyone we saw looked so old and so ill. The majority of the residents were slumped in chairs sleeping, dribbling, or both. My mum was 71, but she looked young for her age and had a lot of energy. How could I bring her here?

My positivity was fading by the minute as I began to consider if we were going to have to find another way to cope. There was no way I could collect Mum from her house and leave her there. I felt bad enough about her situation as it was, but how could I leave her there overnight when I wanted to get out after just ten minutes?

We left feeling very disheartened. Despite how desperate we were, maybe the idea of respite care wasn't such a good one after all.


*24ᵗʰ October, 2017*

To: Cassie and Sam
From: Dad
*Thanks for sorting out the visit and coming over today. I*

*thought the facilities seemed ok. But I would find it hard to send mum there with what we saw of the age and lack of mobility of the residents!*

*I know we don't have anything to judge it by, but it didn't get me excited, if that's the right way to describe the way I felt?*

*Perhaps another care home might? But then we still have to get it right as to how we get mum there!!!*

*Dad xx*


*24th October, 2017*

From: Cassie
To: Dad and Sam
*I agree, I was a bit shocked at how old and ill the majority of the residents looked.*

*I've found two more homes that I will call tomorrow.*

*x*


*25th October, 2017*

To: Dad and Sam
From: Cassie
*Hi Dad and Sam,*

*I've phoned round some more care homes today, I've added the links below, so I don't phone the same ones back. Two of them have a minimum of two weeks, and one of them has a minimum of a one-week stay.*

*I know this isn't ideally what you wanted, Dad, but it*

seems the bigger ones have a minimum stay. Do you think it's worth going to look at the one called Country Court Care?

Another option is that we could look into the care agency staying at your house for a night and you could stay in a hotel/B&B for the night? If that worked, we could look into booking more nights? I know it's not ideal but none of the situations are ideal, and it seems we don't have a lot of choice.

We have had lots of obstacles so far and we didn't know how Mum was going to react until we tried, so I guess it's the same here.

I am out for the day tomorrow but can make some more calls on Friday, unless you get a chance if Mum goes out tomorrow, Dad?

Let me know what you think,

Cassie x

*27th October, 2017*

To: Dad and Sam
From: Cassie
*Hi Dad and Sam,*

*A lady called Laura just called back from the care home called Country Court Care. I said we were a bit hesitant as their minimum stay is one week, but she spent about fifteen minutes going through all of my reservations. She gave me examples of other residents who said they wanted to go home or didn't want to go to bed, and said if they don't want to go to bed, they don't have to as they have 24/7 care.*

*She asked if I'd ask you to give her a call to answer any initial questions you have, and said that we are welcome to visit. I said you wouldn't have a chance until tomorrow.*

*She said they have had a few incidents of people who had to go into care, but didn't get the care home they wanted as it was a rushed decision. She said it is a lot more stressful and more upheaval for everyone, so it's much better to plan in advance and make sure it is the right home.*

*I think it's worth going over to have a look, let me know what you think.*

*Cassie x*

# Chapter Nine

I had only spoken to Laura on the phone once, but for the first time since I could remember, I'd been given a much-needed glimmer of hope. I had almost ended our conversation when she said Mum would have to stay for a whole week. Dad was still so apprehensive about her staying anywhere, so even two nights felt like a long time, particularly when Mum was still getting stressed when my dad was out of her sight for the two hours when the carers were looking after her. How would we manage to get Mum there? What would we say when we left her there? What if she kicked off and got aggressive because she wanted to go home?

I had to temporarily shut the unanswered questions out of my mind, as I was only days away from publishing my second book, *Rule Your World*. Despite having been through one of the hardest years of my life, I had managed to keep my focus, make sacrifices and was proudly publishing my book on the 1st of November 2017 – only five months after I had started writing it.

I had been feeling frustrated for the last month and had lost some confidence in my work. I remember joking to a few people that, "I wanted to put my manuscript in the bin." Be careful what you wish for, as they say, because my considerate postman actually left the first delivery of my books safely in my recycling bin! Thankfully, they were all intact (and didn't smell!), and I had an overwhelming feeling of pride as I took the first copy out of the box.

Mum and Dad were due to arrive at my house later that afternoon, so I signed the first copy for them and placed it on the table. A few hours later, we were all standing in my kitchen laughing at how my books had ended up in the bin, and I proudly handed them their copy. My dad's face lit up as he told me how proud he was and how he loved the front cover. He then passed it to my mum, who looked me straight in the eye and exclaimed, "Wow, this book looks amazing! Did somebody give it to you?"

Did somebody give the book to me? My mum was holding my book in her hand, yet she did not know that the author, her daughter, was standing in front of her. I knew deep down that my mum was proud of me, but it was so bloody hard that she couldn't tell me. I took a deep breath and walked out of the room with tears in my eyes.

These were the kinds of moments that hurt the most. With my first book, I celebrated with a launch in a local bar. I was initially against the idea, but in hindsight I really enjoyed the evening, sharing my achievement with friends and family. So, with this second one, I kept being asked if I was going to have another book launch. I wasn't. How could I give a talk with my mum standing in front of me, not knowing that I was her daughter?

On the 1st of November, I was speaking at an event during the day and hosting an online book launch in the evening. On the 2nd of November, I was being interviewed on the radio, and on the 3rd of November, Dad and I were going to visit the second care home. I didn't have time to feel sorry for myself.

3rd November, 2017

To: Dad and Sam
From: Cassie
*Hi Dad and Sam,*

*Me and Dad went to see this care home today, it was so much better than the last one. It has more of a hotel feel to it, with a coffee shop and hairdressers. All rooms have en-suites, and outside there is a nice garden area. The lady, Laura, was with us for about an hour and was very reassuring.*

*I think it's fair to say that me and Dad were very impressed and feel a lot more at ease for Mum to stay for a week when Dad feels ready.*

*Dad – I have sent a short e-mail to Laura to thank her for her time today and said we'd be in touch once you're ready to book the assessment.*

*Cassie x*

3rd November, 2017

From: Cassie
To: Laura
*Hi Laura,*

*I wanted to thank you for your time today in showing*

*us around the care home. As you know from when we first spoke, my dad had felt very apprehensive about my mum spending time in respite care, but your friendly and caring approach, combined with your outstanding facilities, has really put both of our minds at ease.*

*Please could you also pass on my thanks to the lady and gentleman we spoke to in the corridor. It meant a lot that they both took the time to speak to us. You all made us feel very welcome. The excellent values of Country Court Care were very apparent and have made a lasting impression.*

*I will speak to my dad about booking an assessment and will look forward to getting back in touch once we're ready to go ahead.*

*Kind regards,*
*Cassie*

(N.B The lady who spoke to us was the manager of the care home, and the gentleman was the company finance director)

# Chapter Ten

One month later, I was continuing to juggle the responsibilities of helping my parents, looking after my children, and still trying to make my business a success. I had jumped through many hoops in the hope that my funding application would be approved, attending many workshops and mentoring sessions, not to mention spending over twenty hours preparing cash flow forecasts and future business projections.

Eventually, I hand-delivered my application, along with a copy of both of my books. I hoped that maybe the adviser, who I felt had wrongly judged my business, could understand why it had taken longer than anticipated to increase my profit and turnover. Surely my tenacity and determination to build a business against all the odds counted for something?

I couldn't believe my eyes when a week later I received an e-mail to say that my application had been successful! At last! I could finally invest in the PR and marketing that my business badly needed. I could promote my new book, get my workshops off the ground, and – fingers crossed – get some more bookings as a speaker! It was time for a happy dance around my kitchen, followed by a celebratory cup of tea! They believed in me and they believed in my business. After what had been such a difficult year, I felt the fog lift. Maybe 2018 was going to be the year when everything changed!

*1ˢᵗ December, 2017*

> From: Cassie
> To: Dad
>
> *I got my funding agreement through today with a fifteen-page, very long-winded contract. I've read through the small print and they expect me to pay for all of the costs upfront, not on a credit card, then I have to send them in loads of paperwork. They then have to agree the claim and, if they do, they'll send the money back to me within 30 days.*
>
> *Is there a brick wall nearby I can bash my head against? Surely if I had that money in my account to begin with, I wouldn't be applying for funding in the first place!*
>
> *There are also loads of clauses about how you have to send them financial reports every three months and they have to regularly monitor your outputs, if anything in the contract is breached then you have to repay the money!*
>
> *I won't be going ahead, and I'm not happy that I have wasted days of my time on my application/workshops/ mentoring that I started in August. I've asked why no-one explained the full process to me upfront, I've got no reply.*
>
> *Cassie x*

It felt like things were going from bad to worse in my

business, and the same could be said about the deterioration in Mum's condition. I wasn't looking forward to Christmas. All I wanted was for my mum to be safe, my dad to have a rest – and if my business could succeed, that would be an added bonus!

*26th December, 2017*

From: Cassie
To: Dad
*Hi Dad,*

*I enjoyed our meal today, but it was a shame to see Mum so quiet and confused, I think the noise of the restaurant and busyness was too much for her.*

*After what you said today with Mum going to bed at 4am, soaking the bathroom by flooding the bath, sleeping in her clothes, and making a cup of tea in the kettle, I think we either need to look into some new tablets or go ahead with the respite care.*

*I know we have concerns about the options, but I don't think you can go on indefinitely with the way things are. Mum now seems at risk of something happening.*

*I'm sorry that it feels like I'm the one who is trying to move things forward, but I would rather be proactive. We know that things can change at any time, and it will be me and you who are picking up the pieces.*

*I hope you get a better night's sleep tonight.*

*See you Friday x*

*26th December, 2017*

From: Dad
To: Cassie
*Hi Cassie,*

*Don't be sorry, Cassie, as you know I need a "kick" to get me moving and I am very grateful for all you do/suggest, and as you say something has got to change. If we can just get over New Year and then start planning?*

*See you Friday. x*

*30th December, 2017*

From: Dad
To: Cassie and Sam
*Hi Sam & Cassie,*

*Just to let you know what's been happening over Christmas.*

*Mum's had a few wobbles, for three nights she wouldn't get undressed to go to bed, just slept in her clothes. On Xmas Eve she first mentioned going to bed at 9.20pm, we eventually went to bed at 2am but Mum wanted the bedroom light left on. I got to sleep about 4am, Mum woke me up at 6am, she then went back to sleep, I didn't.*

*Most nights, Mum wants to know where her mum has gone to and when she is coming back, usually I can sort that, but sometimes Mum cries for a while.*

*After talking to Cassie over Christmas, I decided to cancel the companion carers. The lady I spoke to was very understanding. I told her it was nothing to do with the* company or the companions, just Mum's stressed reactions before and long after their visits.

Cassie is going to come over every Friday at the moment to be with Mum for a few hours to give me a break and to get Mum out for the walks I can't do, or just have a wander around the town.

In the New Year we will have to try to sort out some respite care so that I can get some rest. Not sure how that will be done/received, but I'm sure we will sort something out?

If possible, I would like to keep Mum off any more tablets as she doesn't like taking any tablets, but if that's what needed then that's another challenge for me to get over.

Mostly, during the day, Mum is okay and we can do things to keep her active, but it's still the evenings that cause more of a problem and that's when I'm running out of steam!! I find it hard to motivate myself.

I hope that you all have a great New Year and we can meet all the challenges that I'm sure will be just around the corner?

Dad x

31st December, 2017

From: Cassie
To: Dad and Sam

It's sad to hear of Mums decline, but considering it was almost a year ago she was seriously ill in hospital, we have been fortunate to have had another year together, even if there have been a lot of challenges.

*I think the respite care should be a priority and I'm happy to do all of the organising and be the one to take Mum there, if it helps. I think it would do both of you the world of good. From what Laura has said, everyone who has gone there has been fine, no matter how hard it was for the family or the reservations they had.*

*Like we said before, it won't be worse than when Mum was in hospital, and we all survived that.*

*I think if the roles were reversed, Mum would be making these same decisions. It's not nice but I don't feel she's safe longer-term staying at home.*

*I'll call you tonight, Dad.*

*x*


5*th* *January, 2018*

From: Cassie
To: Laura
*Hi Laura,*

*I came and had a look around the home with my dad at the end of last year, with a view to my mum having a week's respite care. My dad has now agreed that he is ready to book the assessment.*

*I will give you a call next week to have a chat to find out what the next step is.*

*Kind regards,*
Cassie


Damn! It was hard to press the *send* button. Yes, it is what I had wanted for months, but it didn't make it any easier. My mum was declining by the day, and my dad was becoming more exhausted. Things had gradually been getting worse, and the carer visits had been causing more stress than they were meant to be reducing. Before the carer arrived, my mum would become stressed, and after they left my mum would become stressed, leaving Dad with more turmoil than he started with.

The last straw was when my mum became aggressive with one of the carers. Apparently, she had stormed out of the house saying that she didn't need a babysitter, and proceeded to swear at the carer in the street!

I was horrified to hear this. This did not sound like my mum – the kind, caring, and compassionate lady who wouldn't hurt a fly. But she knew deep down that something was wrong, she was scared, lost between worlds and neither being here nor there.

# Chapter Eleven

I was already juggling a lot but couldn't bear to see my dad suffering with no real break. So, I offered to start caring for my mum every Friday. This would solve the problem of having strangers in the house, as she kept saying I was the only person she trusted. It also meant that my dad could have longer than two hours to himself and not have to worry about the stressful aftermath once I had left.

*5th January, 2018*

*From: Cassie*

*To: Dad and Sam*

*I managed to have a chat with Dad on Monday, and we've agreed to contact the care home to book an assessment for Mum to have a week's break.*

*This week hasn't been good as I've had bad tonsillitis, so I've been in bed most of the week and not been able to give Dad a break. Mum hasn't been sleeping well, so Dad has not really had a rest.*

*All being well, I will be going over on Sunday. I*

*e-mailed Laura earlier today, saying I'll call her early next week.*

*I'll keep you posted. x*

## 11ᵗʰ January, 2018

> To: Laura
> From: Cassie
> Hi Laura,
>
> It was good to speak to you earlier, thank you for booking my mums assessment for tomorrow. I have completed as much of the form as I can and attached it, I hope that helps.
>
> I am going to collect my mum and take her out for lunch, and then I'll say that you've asked us to meet you for a cup of tea after.
>
> Fingers crossed it all goes ok! See you tomorrow.
> Kind regards,
> Cassie

Oh, my God. This is happening! I'm taking my mum to the care home for an assessment tomorrow, and I feel so apprehensive. I'm scared that she will suspect it's a residential home. What am I going to say if she gets angry and demands to know why she is there? I know it's just an assessment, but the next time we go, I'll be leaving her there for a whole week. Can I really do this?

Laura has been so reassuring and promised that she will do whatever she can to make Mum feel at ease. She even asked me what Mum's favourite biscuits are, and she'll have them ready with a pot of tea. How lovely is that! I have to trust that everything will work out okay.

## 12th January, 2018

"Oh, Cassie! What a lovely surprise, I didn't know you were coming here today."

"I thought I'd come and take you out for the afternoon, Mum. Let's go to the garden centre for lunch. A little bird told me they serve your favourite meal today, fish and chips."

"That sounds lovely. Let me get my bag."

It took me another half an hour to get my mum out of the house, as she needed to check her bag about twenty times, asked numerous questions about where we were going, then check her bag another ten times. I kept my voice calm throughout and reassured her that we'd see my dad again soon.

When we arrived at the garden centre, Mum kept telling me what a lovely time she was having. So far so good. I kept checking the time, and when it was time to leave, I told her that my friend Laura had sent a message to ask if we'd like to meet her for a cup of tea. My mum loves a cup of tea, and told me that sounded like a good plan. It was the next part that I was not looking forward to.

As we drove to the care home, I needed a distraction to keep my nerves at bay and to try and keep Mum as calm as possible. Instinctively, I put on her favourite CD, played her favourite song, *Dancing Queen*, and turned it up... loud!

It worked. By the time we pulled into the car park, my mum was still relaxed.

"Come on, let's go and meet my friend Laura for a cup of tea."

I led Mum towards the front door, knowing this was the moment of truth. I smiled at the receptionist, told her who I was, and that I'd brought my mum to have a cup of tea with *my friend* Laura.

"Hello, yes of course," the lady said. "You've come to join us for a cup of tea today. We've even got your favourite biscuits, custard creams."

Mum's face lit up. "Wow, really, for me? I've come here to teach. I wasn't expecting any biscuits," she replied.

Oh. My. God. I had to stop myself from hugging the receptionist! She had no idea how much her kind welcome meant. I had been dreading this moment for so long, and with just one sentence she had blown away my fears. She not only knew who we were and had gone along with our secret plan, but she had also mentioned the custard creams which was the icing on the cake!

We were then joined by Laura, who greeted my mum by name and told us how much she was looking forward to having a cup of tea and a chat. We went to the coffee shop, where Laura proceeded to make us a lovely pot of tea served in very posh cups and saucers. My mum was in her element and kept thanking me for bringing her for such a lovely day out!

I had asked Laura to be as discreet as possible with her assessment questions, due to Mum's increasing paranoia, and true to her word it was as though we were all having a relaxed chat. I stayed as quiet as I could so that Laura could gauge my mum's capacity.

When Laura was asking Mum questions about her

children, it was obvious that she had no idea that one of them was sitting next to her. At one point, she declared that my sister had met her husband on a bus (she didn't), and that she didn't have any grandchildren (she does). But I sat back, nodded, and smiled in all the right places. As long as my mum felt relaxed, that was all that mattered. Towards the end of the assessment, Laura asked my mum what music she liked and I mentioned that we had played *Dancing Queen* in the car. Well, that was the only cue Mum needed! She started to sing *Dancing Queen* at the top of her voice in the coffee shop. So, what did Laura and I do? We joined in, of course! Then we went back to the reception area, still singing, where my mum thanked the receptionist and Laura, and told them that she'd be back to teach again soon!

As I drove Mum home, I couldn't believe how well our visit had gone. There had been so much that had the potential to go wrong, but it had all turned out so well. The glimmer of hope that Laura had first given me was now a beacon of hope. For the first time since this awful dementia journey began, I finally felt as though we had some support.

# Chapter Twelve

*22<sup>nd</sup> January, 2018*

From: Cassie
To: Dad and Sam
*Hi Dad and Sam,*

*Laura will be back in work on Tuesday and has asked me to call her. I am guessing she will want to know do we have any further questions, and letting me know when they have a space for Mum to visit for a week.*

*I feel that Mum has declined again since Christmas. She seems very anxious, withdrawn, and scared a lot of the time, and isn't able to hold much of a conversation that makes sense. From what Dad is saying, it seems like there are more bad nights than good.*

*With getting Mum to the care home, I will take her for lunch again before saying that we're meeting my friend for a cup of tea.*

*Dad could pack her bag, arrive separately, and unpack it with one of the carers before he leaves.*

*Once I've arrived and had a cup of tea with Mum, I will get up, say that I'm going to find the bathroom, and leave once she is settled.*

*It's obviously not ideal, but Mum was extremely happy last time and didn't know who I was half of the time anyway. I have been reading some advice online and they say not to take a coat or handbag in, so when I leave the table there is no obvious sign that I'm leaving.*

*I can ask Laura what they need packing in the bag, and if they recommend taking some photos, etc, to put in Mum's room.*

*If either of you have any questions, let me know – or if you'd prefer to speak to Laura, Dad, you could call on Thursday when you come here or Friday when I come to your house.*

Let me know what you think. x


*25th January, 2018*

From: Cassie
To: Dad and Sam

*I have just spoken to Laura who said they have had an increase in people wanting to book in, she has eight people to call back today who are in similar situations to us.*

*They can book Mum in on the 1st of February for a week, or the 8th of February for a week.*

*Which one would you prefer, Dad? I am free both days to take Mum and Laura has agreed that you could arrive before with a bag, so I don't have to take that in with Mum.*

*Laura will also send me a checklist of items to pack which you could begin to prepare whilst I take Mum out on the next few Fridays.*

*I'll see you later today, Dad, but as we may not get a*

*chance to speak, I have put all of the information on here.*

*Laura agreed that Mum seemed settled and said she knew it was hard when Mum was speaking to me as if she didn't know who I was. It wasn't nice but I have to see the positive that hopefully Mum won't have the awareness that I will be leaving.*

*Laura has said that you can call her today or tomorrow to have a chat or ask any more questions.*

*She also said that she wanted to pre-warn us that it is becoming common for people who go in for respite care to turn into full-time residents quicker than their carers anticipated. This is because they settle so well into the home and feel safe in the environment that going back to their home can unsettle them. She said that everyone is different, and obviously our first step is to get Mum there and make sure she is happy, but she wanted to mention it.*

*Is there anything new that Mum could do with like a dressing gown/pyjamas etc? We were looking at some clothes today, but she is always very reluctant to buy anything and kept saying she'll see what's left after payday!*

*Maybe start making a list of items like photos/Mum's favourite mug, etc, so it's not a rush on the day.*

*I'll e-mail Laura back and ask if Mum can take a hairdryer. Does Mum keep all her makeup in a bag, as she'll want that, too?*

*Let me know what date you'd prefer and if you want to call or if you want me to x*

*Cassie x*

My mum is now booked in for a week's respite care on the 8th of February. I'm dreading it.

*29ᵗʰ January, 2018*

From: Cassie
To: Dad and Sam
*Hi Dad and Sam,*

*How was Mum after I spoke to her on the phone last night? When I called, Mum cried down the phone for a long time. She couldn't explain herself very well but kept saying she missed her family, she said she keeps on getting a rush of emotion and she can't control it.*

*Unfortunately, this seems to be happening more when I speak to her on the phone. I always try and get her talking and calmed down before I go. I've sent some Reiki this morning and hope that helps.*

*Cassie x*

*29ᵗʰ January, 2018*

From: Dad
To: Cassie and Sam
*Hi Cassie & Sam,*

*After you phoned, Mum stopped crying, and about fifteen minutes later she was calm. She just says how much she misses her family. I try to get her to remember the fun times she had with them which eventually works most times!*

*Mum seems ok this morning, just having her bath before we pop to the coffee shop.*

*Dad x*

*1st February, 2018*

"Oh, wow, Cassie! I didn't know you were coming to see me today. What a lovely surprise, but nobody told me."

"I thought I'd come and see you, Mum. Maybe we could go for a walk and have some lunch in the town."

This was the cue for my dad to say that his leg was playing up and did we mind if he didn't join us.

As always, it took me a long time to get my mum out of the house as she needed to check her bag, ask her questions, and then check her bag another ten times. As always, I kept my voice calm, and reassured her that we'd see my dad again soon.

We began to walk across the park before the questions started. "Where did you grow up? Where did you go to school? Do you have children? Do you take all your friends out for walks?"

I told love lie after love lie, but inside my heart was breaking. We walked around the park, had some lunch in town, then walked back around the park to go home. My mum had been fairly upbeat on the way there but as soon as we began to walk home, I could feel she was starting to become anxious. She started walking at a snail's pace, about three feet behind me. If I stopped walking, she would stop walking. As we got closer to the house, the questions started again. "Where are you taking me? Are they going to take me away? Where's my mum? Does she know where we are? Does she know what time we will be back? Does your mum know where you are? Have you seen my mum today? Is she dead?"

How the hell are you meant to answer these questions?

We got back into the house and I tried to calm her down with as many love lies as I could muster, but nothing was working. While I left the room to make us 'a nice cup of tea', she paced up and down the lounge before sitting like a scared child, repeating the same questions over and over. I tried to distract her by putting on some music and changing the subject, but she wasn't having any of it. Once again, despite not having capacity, she sensed that something was wrong.

"Sit down now! Look me in the eye and promise me that you will never, ever, put me in a care home," she demanded. "I would rather die than be left in an institution. Tell me you would never do that. You are the only person I trust, Cassie. Swear on my life that you will never leave me there. Please, *please,* you have to promise me!"

I held back my tears, knowing that I was about to tell the biggest lie of my life to the woman that I loved the most. Somehow I looked her straight in the eye, then replied, "I promise you, Mum, I will never do that."

# Chapter Thirteen

*February 8, 2018*

After many miles of driving and a flood of memories later, I arrived at my parents' house. Despite the day not starting well, I was surprised at how calm I felt. *You can do this, Cassie, you have dealt with every other challenge life has thrown at you.*

I tried to drown out the millions of 'what ifs' and made-up scenarios that my brain had no answers to. *It's just for one week, she's going to be okay.*

The plan was to get into the house, get my mum ready, and get out of the house asap. The plan was *not* to walk in to find Mum sitting on the sofa, inconsolable. My dad looked up at me with dismay. "Your mum is feeling worried that something bad is going to happen today."

I took a deep breath, sat down next to her, and tried as hard as I could to make my words sound as comforting as possible. "Nothing bad is going to happen today, Mum. I thought we could go to your favourite garden centre and get some lunch. They'll have fish and chips today, as it's Friday. That will be nice, won't it?"

It took another twenty minutes to calm my mum down and convince her that we were going to the garden centre, which – to be fair – was true. I was then going to announce that my friend Laura had text me and asked if we'd like to meet her for a cup of tea, which was also true. I just wasn't going to reveal that the cup of tea would take place in the care home where she would be staying for the next week! My heart hurt with every love lie that was coming out of my mouth, but what else could I do? It was too late to change anything now; Laura was expecting us at 1pm.

I hoped that playing my mum's favourite song in the car would help to ease her worry, but instead of singing along she quietly stared out of the window. By the time we arrived at the garden centre, I had lost track of the amount of times she had asked me where we were going and where my dad was. I replied over and over that we were going out for lunch, Dad was at the coffee shop, and that we would see him later.

When we sat down in the restaurant, things went from bad to worse and she started crying again. I asked her why she was feeling sad, but she found it hard to explain. She kept on telling me that she didn't do it, she didn't mean to hurt anyone, did they get her, and would she be safe?

I am normally good with making up answers, but this was hard work. I had no idea what she was talking about, and no distraction techniques seemed to be working. She kept on asking me why everyone was looking at her, and did they all know? My head was spinning by this point, but I reassured her that everyone was safe, and that no-one was looking at her. I got the impression that she thought she had caused an accident and that a girl on a bike had been hurt.

I tried my best to change the subject and to keep her

calm, but it was challenging in such a busy and noisy environment. By the time we had finished eating and got back to the car, I already felt washed-out. I got my phone out and told my mum that my friend Laura had invited us for a cup of tea and that we were going to meet her now. I started the engine and once again turned up *Dancing Queen* in the hope that it would reduce Mum's anxiety. I had no idea how I would cope if we arrived at the care home with her in tears. If that happened, there was a strong chance that I would also break down, and that wasn't an option.

By some miracle, the music seemed to work and when we pulled into the car park my mum seemed a bit calmer. Once again, the friendly receptionist welcomed Mum by her name, while she declared that she was there to teach some more children! She must have had some recognition of our first visit, as Mum happily greeted Laura and chatted away as we made our way to the lounge area.

We sat down with a cup of tea and it dawned on me that the time had almost come for the part I was not looking forward to. It wasn't long before I would have to get up, leave her there, and walk out. As if right on cue, another gentleman from the home came and sat down with us and told us that he used to be in the navy. When he shared that he had served in Singapore, I almost leapt up and did a dance for joy! My mum had lived in Singapore when she was growing up, and some of her favourite childhood stories that she liked to share (and repeat) were from this time. Hallelujah! Maybe this was going to be okay.

After thirty minutes I gave Laura the nod that I was going to leave, and she asked my mum if she'd like to see where the bathroom was. When my mum agreed and stood up, I knew that was my signal to leave. I watched her walk out of the lounge, said a silent prayer she would be okay, and went to wait in the reception area.

I'd done it! I sat down with a big sigh of relief and hoped that my mum was okay upstairs. In the last ten minutes before I'd left, my mum had been talking to me as if I was a teacher from her old school. It was hard when this happened, but that day I took it as a reassuring sign. My mum wouldn't be upset that her daughter had left, because she didn't know that her daughter had been there.

I waited for Laura to join me once Mum was settled. We had agreed in advance that she would show Mum her own bathroom, which was in her bedroom. My dad had already unpacked her belongings, put up some photos of the family, and positioned her favourite teddy bear on her bed. *Please let her be okay.*

To my relief, Laura walked into the reception with a big smile on her face. She told me that my mum had walked into her bedroom said, "Well, me and my husband must have stayed here before as some of our belongings are here!" She then walked into the lounge where they had *Mamma Mia* playing on DVD (arranged especially for my mum) and she started singing, before sitting down with two other ladies and said, "Hello, how long are you staying at the hotel for?"

That was all I needed to hear. I could finally relax a bit now that I felt reassured that Mum was as settled as she could be. I needed to trust that she was in safe hands now, and let the carers do their job. I would be back to collect her in one week's time.

I sent a message to my dad and my sister to say that,

despite the day not starting well, thankfully Mum had settled in okay and had already made some friends.

I started my drive home feeling shattered, but relieved that it had gone as well as it could have. I would have loved to have gone home, put my pyjamas on, and poured myself a glass of wine. What actually happened was that I went home, gave Kieron some medicine, before racing to the station to catch a train to London for a meeting! Returning home at 10pm was far from ideal, but my life had to go on, despite putting my mum's needs first.

# Chapter Fourteen

We had been advised not to visit Mum during her stay, so that she could fully settle into her new routine and so that Dad could have a much-needed rest. I was so happy when my dad told me he was going to have a break away for a few days. Before my mum's condition had worsened, my parents had frequently gone for weekends away, but this had become a distant memory – as had a full night's sleep. We decided that he would go away for the first three nights and that I would be on 'standby' just in case anything happened and we needed to get to the care home. Then I would take the boys away for a night and my dad would stay close by for the last two days. Dad understandably felt apprehensive, but he was also looking forward to the simple things like reading, having a coffee, or an afternoon nap, without constantly being on high alert.

We both enjoyed our time away, and before we knew it, it was time to begin 'operation bring mum home'. The plan was that I would go and collect her, take her out for lunch while Dad collected her belongings and took them home. This meant that when we arrived home, everything would be there and we 'hoped' that she wouldn't know she'd ever been away.

I felt apprehensive walking back into the care home, not knowing how my mum would be. The carers told me that she had settled after a couple of days, but that she hadn't been to bed a couple of nights. One of those nights she had sat up all night with another lady 'having a meeting'! Apparently, they were planning a new company!

I walked into the lounge and found her asleep in a chair, snoring. When she woke up, she didn't seem 'with it' at all. She asked a few questions about where her mum was, but mainly she was in a daze. Part of me didn't want to take her back home. Maybe as she had lived in a safe environment, she had stopped fighting her condition and had allowed herself to rest?

I linked my arm through hers and walked out to the car. She moved in slow motion, got into the car, and fell back to sleep. As we got closer to the garden centre, I decided to just carry on driving. It was a bit like if you wake a baby up when they are fast asleep, you know you're asking for trouble. So, I decided to keep on driving in the hope that when she finally did wake up, she'd be a bit more alert.

When we reached my mum and dad's town, she was still fast asleep, so I carried on driving for another 10 miles. I then turned around to drive back to find somewhere to eat, where I waited for the text to say Dad had collected her belongings and had arrived back home.

Once we had finished our lunch, I received the message from my dad. The final step was to hope that Mum was oblivious to her week away. She walked into the house and immediately asked my dad where he had been. But when he replied that he'd been to the coffee shop, she simply sat down, closed her eyes, and slept for the rest of the day. Mission accomplished.

I felt so relieved that what had started out as a very daunting task had been such a success. I wish the same could be said about my business.

The words of the business adviser still rang in my ears, "Why do you think your business hasn't been successful? Do you really believe you have what it takes to make this work?" If only he could have been a fly on the wall for the last six months to see the many challenges I'd faced. But was I putting too much pressure on myself to run a business when my family needed so much support?

Whenever I've hit a brick wall in the past, there has often been a little glimmer of hope as if to say, "Don't give up." It might have been a new book review, a speaking opportunity, or a message to say how I've inspired or helped someone.

After a very dark few months, my glimmer of hope this time came in the form of a message from Estelle Keeber and Leona Burton, the founders of MIBA (Mums in Business Association)

Estelle & Leona: *Hey, Cassie, we were wondering if you'd like to run a Facebook live in our group?*

Cassie: *I'd love to, what would you like me to speak about?*

Estelle & Leona: *We'd love you to speak about how to write a book.*

How to write a book? Could I do that? Did I have enough content to share?

Cassie: *Yes, I'd love to. Let's get a date booked in!*

Talk about stepping out of your comfort zone? This was more like a bungee jump! Yes, I had written two books, but I honestly wasn't sure if I could speak for an hour on the topic! Well, I would soon find out!

I wrote out my notes and hoped for the best.

Oh, my goodness, I did it! I don't know what I had been worrying about. I spoke in the Mums in Business Association Facebook group, which has over 10,000 members and could not believe the positive response I got. I received so many messages from people telling me how much my story had inspired them, that they had never thought it was possible to write a book but now they believed they could.

*Facebook message*

From: Lyndsey
To: Cassie
*Hi Cassie,*

*I stumbled across your video today in the Mums in Business Association group about writing a book. This is something I've toyed with for over a year but thought nobody would want to hear what I have to say. I just wanted to say a huge THANK YOU!! Your video gave me whatever it was I needed to put pen to paper and get my ideas down.*

*Just in case nobody has told you today, you're an absolute inspiration.*

*Thank you again for taking the time to make the video, you've probably helped more people than you realise.*
*Lyndsey x*

There were also people asking me if I offered author mentoring. Err, give me a few days and I will! Maybe this was the path that had been waiting for me all along. When I wrote my first book, *The Girl Who Refused to Quit*, I had no idea how powerful it would be. I didn't know that it would form a huge part of my healing journey and that it would enable me to make peace with my past. What if I could help other people to write a book that would support them to heal and release their past?

For the first time for as long as I could remember, I felt my soul come alive. I had to be brave and take action before I lost my nerve. I started to brainstorm everything I had learned, and that's when it came to me: I should write a book on how to write a life-changing book.

I took a huge leap of faith and invested in working with a new coach, Lauren Robertson, who immediately told me that I should create an author mentoring programme and begin to work with clients right now. Right now? Surely, I should write my book and then gain some clients once people knew about my work? Her response? "Cassie, you have published two books, you are already an expert. I believe in you; it's time for you to believe in yourself. Here's what you're going to do. Write out your programme, create a video to promote your programme, and get to work!"

# Chapter Fifteen

With some much-needed fire in my belly, I did indeed get to work. I wrote out my new programme and set up my video recording equipment. Just as I was about to press *record,* my phone rang. It was Dad. He was due to bring my mum over for a visit that afternoon, but told me that she wasn't having a good day and asked me to speak to her.

My mum tried to speak but couldn't get her words out. Instead, she started to cry her eyes out whilst her increased anxiety caused her to have a panic attack. I tried to calm her down, but nothing was working. She couldn't comprehend the words I was saying, and her anxiety was increasingly causing her to hyperventilate.

I don't know if you can imagine hearing someone you love having a panic attack on the other end of the phone? That on its own was horrific enough, but due to her dementia, nothing I said was being stored in her brain or remembered. She continued to sob and repeat her muttered words over and over. I wanted to cry myself, but continued to reassure her she was safe and, somehow, a good fifteen minutes later, I managed to calm her down. She handed the phone back to my dad who agreed to get her a cup of tea, warm her up, and try again to come over to my house so they could both have a break.

I ended the call and just sobbed my heart out. Why was this bloody condition so cruel? Not only for the person who is suffering, but for all of their loved ones, too. I was trying my goddamned hardest to be there for everyone, whilst trying to build a business so that I could support my family, but I couldn't take much more.

I couldn't record a video for my new mentoring programme with mascara streaming down my face and snot streaming down my nose. But spontaneously, I decided to press record and make a video for my dad and sister instead.

*3rd March, 2018*

From: Cassie

To: Dad and Sam

*Re: Today was the day I cracked*

*As you both know, it's been an extremely difficult few months, but after listening to Mum crying and having a panic attack down the phone today, I cracked. I cried my eyes out, and then had to pull myself together and went on the school run five minutes later.*

*Mum and Dad did end up coming over. Mum had calmed down and we did some gardening, so it all ended well, but I wanted to make a video to show that I'm not always able to be strong.*

*I didn't plan on making a video, but it was all set up to record my new programme, and I wanted to be honest about how I felt. I've added the link below.*

*I hope you get a better sleep tonight, Dad, and that Mum is calmer tomorrow.*

*Cassie x*

As each day passed, the challenges were getting bigger as my mum continued to slip away into another world. I noticed on my visits that having previously walked for three hours, she could now barely walk for twenty minutes without being exhausted.

Despite the heartache of my mum's decline, I somehow managed to pick myself up, launch my programme, plan a live workshop, and continue to write my third book, *Share Your World – How to write a life-changing book in 60 days.*

*25ᵗʰ March, 2018*

From: Cassie

To: Dad and Sam

*I've just had another call with Mum sobbing down the phone, extremely upset and confused asking if her mum was dead.*

*I know Mum still has some happy moments, but I feel we all need to be realistic and recognise that she has a serious condition that is getting progressively worse, which is affecting all of us.*

*We have done our best to care for Mum, but I don't feel we can carry on like this indefinitely.*

*I'm going to be completely honest and say I don't think it's fair on Mum to be living at home any more. She is getting increasingly frail, upset, and anxious. I feel she needs to have 24-hour care.*

*I really hope Mum has been able to calm down and that you are ok, Dad.*

*Cassie x*

# Chapter Sixteen

I t was time to admit that we could no longer provide the level of care that my mum needed. It was time to face the decision that we had all been dreading.

On the 31st of March 2018, my dad made that heartbreaking decision.

*27th April, 2018*

It felt like *déjà vu* as I got into my car, turned the music up, and prayed that I could get through the day without breaking down. I arrived at my parents' house hoping that Mum wouldn't be crying again. *Please don't be crying.* I was shocked to walk in to find her smiling and ready to go! Her shoes were on, her coat was on, and she got up and gave me a big hug. "Hello, Sunshine, I'm so happy you've come to see me today. Are we going to go out?" I had to look away from my dad as the realisation of what was happening kicked in.

"Hi Mum, that's right," I answered brightly. "I thought we could go to our favourite place for lunch and maybe meet my friend Laura for a cup of tea after?"

In all honesty, I don't know what was worse: collecting

my mum when she was inconsolably crying, or collecting her when she was upbeat and happy. She was totally oblivious to the fact that once she said goodbye to her husband and walked out the door, she would never return to the home where they had lived together for the last 30 years.

I'm not sure how I held it together, but I managed to give my dad a quick smile, and told him we'd '*see him later*', as we got into the car.

I put all my emotions to one side and kept as calm and as positive as possible. I knew my mum would pick up on my anxiety if I fell to pieces. I had hoped that we could have a short walk before lunch, but the torrential rain had scuppered those plans. By the time we sat down for our lunch, Mum was already speaking to me as if I was someone else, which I was grateful for. It hurt that she thought I was her friend from London, but it gave me the reassurance that it would be easier to leave her if she didn't know who I was.

I kept a close eye on the time, counting down the minutes before we had to leave for the next part of our journey. Despite not making a lot of sense, Mum was surprisingly upbeat and remained positive when I told her that we were going to meet my friend Laura for a cup of tea.

I started the engine, turned up *Dancing Queen* as loud as I could bear, and we sang our hearts out all the way until we reached the car park of where she'd be living from then on. This was it; no going back now.

I looked anxiously across at my mum, but to my surprise she had a huge smile on her face. "Wow, this place looks lovely, are we going to go in?"

For once, I didn't have to lie. "Yes, we are going in. Let's go and meet my friend Laura."

My mum got out of the car with a spring in her step. "Thank you so much for bringing me here. I've had such a lovely day with you." She had no idea that once she stepped into the care home, she would be spending the rest of her life there... and for that I was grateful.

Once again, we received a warm welcome from Laura who introduced us to Jo, the main carer who would be looking after my mum. Jo spent the next hour talking to Mum and asking her questions. My mum very convincingly gave all of the 'wrong' answers but, as always, I didn't interrupt or correct her. I didn't even flinch when she spoke about her daughter Cassandra who didn't have any children; all that mattered was that Mum felt like she was in control.

There was a slight blip when Jo asked my mum if she remembered staying there before, to which she replied, yes. I knew she didn't really remember staying, but Mum often said yes to questions because she didn't want anyone to think that she couldn't remember something. Jo was oblivious to this, so then asked my mum if she'd like to look at her room. At this point, Mum panicked. She asked why she needed a room when she wasn't staying there. She asked where my dad was, and then turned to me and said, "You're not leaving me here, are you?" My stomach lurched in panic. *Oh, my goodness, help me, please somebody help me!*

I put on my best reassuring voice and told Mum that we wouldn't be staying there as neither of us had brought any bags with us. I explained that what Jo really meant to say was that she would show her where the bathroom was. Thankfully, this managed to relax her. My mum didn't know who I was, but she still trusted me enough to stand up and follow Jo to the bathroom. I knew that this was my cue to leave.

I wanted to give Mum a hug, tell her that I loved her and that I'd see her again soon, but this wasn't about me and my needs. I had to do what was right for her, which was to leave her in the hands of the staff who would be keeping her safe from that moment on. As soon as they walked out of the lounge, I went back to the reception area and waited to hear that she had settled in and that it was okay for me to leave.

I expected to be consumed by a huge amount of guilt as I sat and waited. But as I took a moment to relive what had happened, it took me by surprise at how relieved I felt. Yes, our lives were going to be very different from that moment on, but my mum was safe now. Ten minutes passed before Jo reassured me that Mum was okay and that I could leave. Once again, we were advised not to visit immediately, to allow her time to settle in.

One week later, I walked apprehensively back into the care home, not knowing what to expect. How would Mum react? Would she be angry at me for leaving her there? What would I say if she wanted to go home?

I saw her in the lounge before she saw me. She looked happy, sitting in a chair with a cup of tea, chatting away to some new friends. She caught my eye, gave me a huge smile, stood up, and held her arms out towards me. I made my way across the room towards the big embrace that awaited as my mum joyfully began to speak. "I knew it! I knew you would come. I've been telling everyone about you. Come over and sit down."

Oh, my goodness, what a welcome! I hadn't been expecting this.

"I want to hear all of your news. Tell me, how are you? And how is your mum?"

*How is my mum? Did you actually just ask me how my mum is? I'm your daughter!*

"Err, yeah. I'm okay." *Please let that be a one-off; please do not ask me about my mum again!* I used to feel frustrated that my mum only knew who I was for the first ten minutes of seeing me, but now I was wishing we could go back in time. Had she now completely forgotten who I was?

I wanted to get up and walk out right then and there. What are you meant to do when you want to relinquish all responsibility and run away? The thoughts rushing around my head didn't stop my mum from carrying on with her questions.

"Where is your mum today? What's your mum doing?"

I wanted to shout, "YOU ARE MY MUM!" I've never had any training of how to speak to someone with dementia, but I have learned through experience that you never correct them, you don't raise your voice, and you don't make them feel inferior.

I dug deep for some much-needed strength and forced a calm answer to come out of my mouth. "My mum's at home, she's in the garden."

I must have sounded convincing, as my mum was beaming a huge smile at me whilst her friends were keen to know who her new companion was.

"Who's come to visit you? Is this your daughter?"

"You didn't tell us you had such a beautiful daughter. You look so alike, you can tell that you are both related."

Cue my mum staring into space like someone had told her that an alien had just landed in the lounge.

Confused and still wanting answers, one of my mum's new friends turned to me and asked, "Is she your mum?"

I gave a solemn nod and whispered, "Yes, but she doesn't know who I am." I could feel the sadness building inside me. This wasn't meant to happen. My mum had always known who I was for the first ten minutes. She would usually greet me with a hug and tell me how happy she was to see me. She would always ask how the boys were. She would tell me what an amazing mum I was, and that she was so proud of me. It was only after that she would start to repeat her favourite childhood stories, not speak a lot of sense, and *then* speak to me like I was someone else. Even though it was always hard, I could cope because she knew who I was for those first precious ten minutes.

Where had that time gone? Where had my mum gone?

I'm not sure how I got through the next hour of her relentless questions and my made-up answers. When it was time to leave, I said I was going to find the bathroom, got up, and headed towards my mum's room. That was another tip I had picked up from the online support forum: never say goodbye when you're leaving; and never mention that you're going home. I believed that home was no longer a place for my mum, it was a feeling. Before she lived in the care home, Mum would often cry and say that she wanted to go home, even though she was in her own house. I believe what she really wanted was the feeling which she associated with home, the feeling of being safe.

She felt safe now, so she was home.

# Chapter Seventeen

Anyone who walked into the care home for the first time could easily mistake it for a hotel. The interior decor is high quality, with a warm and welcoming feel. My mum's room was the same. I stepped in and thought how lovely, bright, and clean everything looked, before my eyes caught sight of the photographs on the window sill. For a moment, they took my breath away. Staring back at me were the innocent smiles of my beloved children; my mum's beloved grandchildren. The tears I had fought for the last hour started to fall uncontrollably down my face. It was only ten days since we had all sat around my dining room table, eating pizza and laughing. The boys had said goodbye to their nana, knowing that she was soon to be living in a care home. I had been honest with them and explained that it wasn't safe for Nana to live at home any more, but that they'd be able to visit her once she'd settled in. The last hour had just changed everything.

Was it fair to put the boys through the emotional torment that I had just experienced? What would they say to their nana if she asked them who they were? Could I expect them to compulsively lie and cope with the emotions that came with that? They were 15 and 9 years old, so I would give them the choice and allow them to decide. But as I stood in my mum's bedroom silently sobbing, I had an awful feeling that my children would never see their nana again.

This wasn't meant to happen; it wasn't meant to be this way! How could I explain that they would have to either choose to see their nana, who didn't know who they were, or decide to never see her again? Had they not coped with enough crap in their lives already? How was I meant to handle this situation?

Have you ever had a moment in your life when, out of nowhere, a stranger appears at exactly the right time? I must have been crying louder than I realised, when suddenly I became aware of a lady standing in the doorway of my mum's room. I must have looked like a right state, and wouldn't have blamed her for walking on by. Instead, she gave me a warm smile and said, "Would you like a hug?" Well, that set me off again.

We hugged, spoke, and cried together for the next ten minutes, and she explained that she was going through a similar experience with her mum. There was nothing that she could say or do to change my situation, but knowing that I wasn't going crazy and that I wasn't the only one who felt this way, brought me some much-needed comfort.

I just about managed the drive home without crying, but the same couldn't be said when I had the dreaded conversation with the boys that evening. I could have delayed it for a few days or bent the truth when they asked how Nana was. But as my head already felt like it was going to explode, I decided to bite the bullet and deal with it straight-on.

I can't remember the exact words I said to the boys, but I ended up crying as I explained to them that there was a good chance that Nana would no longer know who they were. I told them that they both had a choice – to visit with the risk of her not knowing who they were, or to not visit and remember the old nana, the way she used to be.

Despite the amount of unexpected challenges my boys have faced in their life, it has never ceased to amaze me how emotionally mature they are, and this situation was no different. They were both very calm and, after thinking about it, they both decided that they wanted to remember Nana the way she used to be.

Part of me was devastated that they would never see her again. Another part of me was relieved that they wouldn't have to endure an upsetting visit. But there was also part of me that was envious. I didn't feel I had the same choice to walk away.

I would continue to visit my mum whether she knew who I was or not, whether I wanted to or not. I would be there and love her unconditionally, no matter what.

# Chapter Eighteen

*December 2018*

*Why do I bother?*

Since the day I left Mum at the care home, she hasn't known who I am. She has moments of remembering my dad, and times when she remembers her friends, but she has completely forgotten me. There have been a few occasions when she tells me about her daughter, Cassie, but most of the time she speaks to me as though I'm one of her friends. Despite how hard this is, I have continued to visit her regularly. There are times when she is awake, confused, and disorientated, other times I arrive to find her fast asleep. Either way, she doesn't know that I have been to see her.

I have been asked several times why I make the journey to see someone who has no recollection of my visit.

I never thought I'd say this, but over time the visits have become easier. I have found that I feel less angry at that way things *should* have been, and have tried to accept them for what they are.

Yes, it hurts that I will never have a *normal* conversation with my mum ever again. It breaks my heart that I will never hear her call me by my name and that I will never call her Mum ever again, but I have to remind myself that, in her own little world, she is safe and happy.

The hardest visit was when I arrived to find her in a really bad mood. It was the day before my birthday, and I had already been feeling low due to one too many 'life challenges' piling on top of me. I also felt sad that it was the first birthday when I wouldn't hear her say "Happy birthday, Sunshine", but still, I wanted to see her.

As always, I took a deep breath, tried to 'leave myself' in the car park, and headed in to find my mum.

I found her pacing the corridor looking really agitated. "Hello," I said with a smile, but she was having none of it.

"Get away from me!" she snarled. She looked me right in the eyes as her anger boiled over. "You don't know me, get out of my way, will you just leave me alone!"

This was the second time I considered walking out. Should I stay or should I go? My emotions were torn. I wouldn't accept this behaviour from anyone else, but she was my mum and deep down I knew she didn't mean to upset me.

I said a quick prayer for help, and five minutes later I had convinced her to sit down in the dining room. She was still looking at me like she hated me, and her face and body were tense. Instinctively, I reached my hands out and asked if I could warm her hands up. As I held Mum's hands, her body instantly relaxed and she closed her eyes. Thank God for that. *You're safe now mum. Please, don't be angry.*

To my complete surprise, she opened her eyes, looked straight into mine, and said, "You are so beautiful. You are such a kind and caring lady. Please don't ever leave me."

Well, that was it. My tears started flowing, and they didn't stop for quite some time. I could see that a lot of the other residents were looking at me and wondering why the new lady was sitting at the dining table in tears, but I couldn't help myself. I heard one of the residents ask her friend why I was crying, and he replied, "That's her mum. You can't imagine how hard it must be to lose your mum and still visit her."

I walked out and into the reception area with tears and mascara streaming down my face. Laura was busy working, but I asked her if I could have a hug. She stopped her work, hugged me, and spoke to me until I was calm enough to drive. Before I left, she admitted, "I did wonder when this was going to happen, you've been so strong for so long." She was right. I had been, but what choice did I have?

My happiest visit was, ironically, on a day I had not looked forward to – Mum's birthday. It was another 'first' that I felt emotional about. I had asked my friend to bake some cakes to take in, and went to collect them from her house with Lennie. On our way home, Lennie asked me, "Mum, are we all taking the cakes to visit Nana tomorrow?" I was gobsmacked. He hadn't seen my mum for four months, after deciding to remember 'the old nana.' I told him that I would love him to visit, but to be prepared for her not knowing who he was or that it was her birthday.

He asked me what the care home was like, and when I said it's like a lovely hotel, he decided to come. I wanted Lennie to see my mum, but at the same time I felt apprehensive and prayed all the way that she wouldn't be angry or upset.

Well, I have never seen my mum in such high spirits!

Her carer had dressed her in a lovely blue dress and arranged for her to go the on-site hairdresser's. Lennie and I took her to the salon whilst we all sang *Happy Birthday*.

We were walking along the corridor singing, when Lennie asked if he could have one of the cakes. "That's fine," I said. "Give me two secs and let's get Nana settled first."

"SEX!" shouted my mum, laughing her head off. "It's a bit early for that!" I was crying with laughter, and quickly passed Lennie a cake so that I didn't have to explain the joke!

The radio in the hairdresser's salon didn't have a great reception, so I asked if I could play my mum's favourite song, *Dancing Queen*. I got my phone out, turned up the volume, and we all sang whilst the hairdresser trimmed my mum's hair.

She was still on a high when we went back to the lounge, and we continued to play *Dancing Queen* on repeat for the next hour whilst we sang and danced together. The joy that was beaming out of my mum was incredible! It was a beautiful moment that I wanted to keep in my heart forever, and thankfully Lennie (the video man) was there to capture it all on my phone.

My mum may not know who I am, but I believe that her soul still recognises mine.

*That* is why I bother.

# Epilogue

*July 16, 2018*

To: Dad and Sam
From: Cassie
*I went to visit Mum today. She was very quiet, and was just saying random words instead of the normal random sentences.*

*I told Laura that I am thinking of writing a book about losing a parent to dementia.*

*Obviously, I need to publish book three first!*

*Cassie x*

*My favourite song Read all about it by Emeli Sandé was playing on the radio as we spoke, maybe that's a sign?!*

*November 1, 2018*

One year to the day since publishing *Rule Your World* against all the odds, I published my third book, *Share Your World – How to write a life-changing book in 60 days.*

Dedicating *Share Your World* to my mum, knowing not only that she will never read it, but that she no longer knows who I am, is simply heart-breaking. This was the message I wrote in my mum's copy of the book: 'To my amazing mum, love from your Sunshine.'

*November 19, 2018*

An extract from a post I wrote in The Unforgettable Dementia Support Facebook group:

> Today I have started to write a book called, *I've Lost My Mum.*
>
> There have been so many times I have felt alone, scared, and isolated on this awful journey, yet despite this, I am constantly told how well I 'cope' with my mum having dementia and no longer knowing who I am.
>
> I am making a commitment to myself and to everyone who needs to read it that this book is happening.
>
> Thank you for providing this safe space.

*December 11, 2018*

An extract from a Facebook post on my profile:

> 28 days.
> 22,282 words.
> Too many tears to count.
> The first draft of my fourth book, *I've Lost My Mum*, is written.

*March 3, 2019*

Writing this book has taken a little longer than I had hoped, as I have now been commissioned to write three books as a soul-writer (a bit like a spiritual ghost-writer). My first clients were Estelle and Leona, the amazing co-founders of Mums in Business Association, who helped me to change the direction of my business last year.

All of our lives have changed so much in such a short space of time, especially my dad's. Despite visiting my mum three times a week, every single week, he still misses her company. He is relieved that she is safe but it's a huge change to make, going from living with someone for forty years to adjusting to life on your own.

I am starting to feel a bit apprehensive about sharing our journey, but I keep reminding myself that I have not come this far only to come this far. I will keep going and I will publish this book.

I was reading through my manuscript for the final time this evening, before sending it to my editor in the morning. I received a phone call from my dad, who told me that he has found Mum's old diary dating back to 2014. My mum never admitted to us that she had dementia. But we now know that in the beginning she knew, and still had a great sense of humour!

This is an extract from her diary:

*November 25, 2014*

*After a long and reassuring visit with Dr_____, I was shocked to hear that I have dementia.*

*I will cope with it, and I refuse to let it get me down. Life is for living so let's get on and do it.*

*It won't be easy, and I know it will be difficult not to want to tear your hair out. Think yourself lucky you haven't got it. Lucky things! Or maybe you are the weirdos and I'm normal!!??*

Unfortunately, there is no happy-ever-after in this book. My mum's condition is continuing to decline.

I honestly didn't know if I'd make it past 237 words, but now that I've reached 27,238, I'm feeling proud that I followed my mum's advice:

*"If you can do something that will help just one person, then I think you should do it."*

Cassandra Farren's amazing mum.

# A poem for my mum

You're not gone, but you're no longer here.
Where is my mum who used to hold me so dear?
Are your memories safely locked away?
Or, like your world, have they started to fade?
Not knowing who I am hurts me for sure,
But I'll stay by your side forever more.
I may have lost you in the way I once knew,
But I will never lose the love I have for you.
Thank you for the laughter, the smiles, and the fun
You are my one and only, very special mum.

# About the Author

Cassandra, who lives in Northamptonshire, England, has been described as "a gentle soul powered by rocket fuel!"

When she's not mentoring authors or writing life-changing books, Cassandra can often be found relaxing by a beautiful lake or having a dance party in her kitchen!

She is a very proud Soul Writer and Reiki Master who has committed to her own journey of personal and spiritual growth.

Cassandra's mission is to create a new generation of heart-led authors who collectively make a difference in the world, one book at a time.

# Top Tips from
# an Admiral Nurse

Admiral Nurse, Caroline Clifton works for Belong and supports carers and families of people with dementia. As a specialist mental health nurse, she helps increase understanding of techniques to support people with dementia.

Here are her top tips for family members and professionals.

1) Get to know the person
   Know their likes and dislikes
   Gather life history
   Have three points of conversation
2) Maintain eye contact and smile!
   The person with dementia will notice;
   Your emotional state
   Your body language
   Tone of voice
3) Slow down
   Provide care in a relaxed manner
   Help the person to do things for themselves
   Keep it simple
4) Introduce yourself every time

Tell the person your name
Tell them what you are there for
Refer to the person by their name

5) Communicate clearly
Talk about one thing at a time
Offer simple choices
Speak clearly in a warm calm voice

6) Step into the person's world
If the person becomes upset
Reassure the person
Acknowledge that you can see the person is upset
Validate what the person is saying or doing

7) Keep it quiet
Create a relaxed environment
Stop, listen and avoid distraction
Reduce conflicting noises
Avoid crowds and lots of noise

8) Don't argue or quibble
Go with the flow
Acknowledge and respect what the person is saying and doing
Telling them they are wrong may have a negative effect

9) Engage and encourage
Get the person started with a meaningful activity
Set activities up to succeed and have fun
Focus on what the person can do

10) Talk with others
Share your experiences with others
Talk together about what has happened and how you coped with the situation
Record what has helped and what has not

*A different reality… becoming a 'dementia detective.'*

Avoid contradicting the person with dementia as this could increase their anxiety. Remember that, at that moment, what they are saying is what they believe to be true as this is the person's reality.

Join their world! Focus on how you can put the person at ease, thus reducing their anxiety.

For example: If the person is always asking for their mother, whom you know is deceased, this can indicate a need for closeness, acceptance, affection or support.

Rather than correcting them, you could simply respond 'Tell me about your mum, what was she like?' or 'Are you feeling upset at the moment?', 'I know I'm not your mum, but is there anything I can do for you?'

A person may believe that they still have a young son and they need to make his tea. This can indicate, for example, a need for being involved in activity that has value or purpose, or the need to feel needed. Try saying 'Have you any photographs of him? I'd like to see them. I bet he was a handful' or simply 'You must be really proud of him.'

A person might, for example, ask to go home during the evening. Try asking 'Do you feel tired?' or 'Do you want to go home so that you can lie down? There is a room here for you with a nice comfy bed. We could go there now so that you can have a rest, would that be ok?'

Do not feel guilty that you are encouraging what may seem to you as fantasy. If you can make the person with dementia feel content, relaxed and at ease rather than anxious, sad or distressed, you are simply doing the best thing for them.

Learn to piece together the phrases, signals and behaviour of the person. Always focus on the emotion, rather than the actual communication. It is better to respond to the person's feelings and try to address their needs.

When you know the meaning behind the behaviour, you'll be more able to find solutions to help the person cope.

The better we know a person, the more we can build up knowledge of what they might need when they say a certain comment or question.

When we build up this awareness of an individual's way of communicating, it not only helps us to find an effective response to a tricky question, it means we can also put plans in place to address the person's needs.

We can then share this plan and knowledge with everyone involved in supporting the person.

With thanks to Caroline Clifton, Admiral Nurse, Belong.

www.belong.org.uk

# Resources

References are provided for informational purposes only and do not constitute endorsement of any websites or other sources. Readers should be aware that the websites listed in this book may change.

A list of resources can also be found at:
www.cassandrafarren.com/ive-lost-my-mum/

*Age UK*
0800 055 6112
www.ageuk.org.uk

*Alzheimer's Society*
www.alzheimers.org.uk

*Alzheimer's Research UK*
www.alzheimersresearch.org

*Carers Trust*
0300 772 9600
www.carers.org

*Care Choices*
01223 207770
www.carechoices.co.uk

*Country Court Care*
Providing residential, dementia and nursing care across the UK.
01733 571951
www.countrycourtcare.com

*Dementia Action Alliance*
www.dementiaaction.org.uk

*Dementia Friends*
www.dementiafriends.org.uk

*Dementia UK*
0800 888 6678
www.dementiauk.org

*National Dementia Helpline*
0300 222 1122

*Unforgettable*
Unforgettable provides a range of dementia products, services and advice to improve the lives of those affected by dementia, Alzheimer's and memory loss.
www.unforgettable.org
www.facebook.com/groups/
UnforgettableDementiaSupport

# The Girl Who Refused to Quit

*The Girl Who Refused to Quit* tells the surprisingly uplifting journey of a young woman who has overcome more than her fair share of challenges.

When she hit rock bottom for the third time Cassandra was left questioning her worth and her purpose. She could have been forgiven for giving up on everything. Instead she chose to transform adversity into triumph and with not much more than sheer determination Cassandra has now set up her own business to empower other women.

She is the girl who refused to be defined by her circumstances. She is the girl who wants to inspire other women, to show them that no matter what challenges you face you can still hold your head high, believe in yourself and follow your dreams.

She is *The Girl Who Refused to Quit*.

# Rule Your World

*Reduce Your Stress, Regain Your Control & Restore Your Calm*

Have you ever questioned why your head is in such a mess – even when your life appears to look so good?

You know something needs to change, but don't know where to start?

When she became a single parent for the third time Cassandra feared her head may become a bigger mess than her life and inadvertently began to follow "The Rules".

Sharing her thought provoking and refreshing personal insights Cassandra's 7 rules will help to raise your self-awareness and empower a calmer, more fulfilling way of living.

Combining relatable real-life stories, and intriguing scientific studies with simple but powerful exercises, you will gain your own "Toolbox for Life" as well as admiration for this determined and strong woman.

Cassandra is living proof that when you reduce your stress, regain your control & restore your calm, you too can Rule Your World.

# Share Your World

*How to write a life-changing book in 60 days*

How many times do you need to be told, "You should write a book" before you finally believe that you could become an author?

Your heart wants to share your story, but your head feels overwhelmed; Where do you find the courage to start, how do you make a plan to ensure you finish, and who would really want to read about your real-life journey?

Cassandra has written a positive and practical guide for aspiring authors, who want to make a difference to the lives of others by sharing their story.

In her natural, relaxed (and brutally honest!) style of writing, Cassandra shares her simple tools and tips whilst letting you into her own inspiring, yet unlikely, story of how she became the author of three books.

Cassandra's uplifting guidance will empower you to Share Your World and write a life-changing book, in only 60 days!

# Contact Cassandra

www.cassandrafarren.com

Register for updates on future books and talks

www.cassandrafarren.com/ive-lost-my-mum/
Facebook/cassandrafarren1
Facebook/groups/heartledauthors
Linkedin/cassandrafarren.com
For mentoring, speaking or press enquiries please e-mail
hello@cassandrafarren.com

Printed in Great Britain
by Amazon

41489181R10076